AF677389

FAITH, FOCUS, AND FULFILLMENT: YOUR GUIDE TO CONQUERING THE AGPCNP EXAM WITH GRACE.

A STEP-BY-STEP GUIDE

LOVE CHRISTOPHERS

CONTENTS

FOREWORD

Faith, Focus, and Fulfillment: A Guide to Conquering the AGPCNP Exam with Grace

Welcome to the foreword of the guide that aims to help you prepare for the Adult Gerontology Primary Care Nurse Practitioner (AGPCNP) exam. Success requires dedication, focus, and a strong belief in your abilities. As you hold this book, *Faith, Focus, and Fulfillment: Your Guide to Conquering the AGPCNP Exam with Grace*, you are taking a crucial step toward achieving your goal—not just to pass an exam, but to fulfill your calling to serve and heal as a compassionate caregiver.

This guide, authored by Love Christophers, an experienced AGPCNP student with years of clinical practice and academic knowledge, is the culmination of her personal experiences, dedicated study, prayer, and unwavering determination. *This guide is designed to complement and enhance the invaluable lessons and clinical knowledge you have gained in nursing school.* Rather, it serves as a companion—a tool to refine your focus, inspire your faith, and solidify your knowledge as you prepare for this important milestone. The insights, notes, and strategies in these pages, including detailed study schedules, real-life clinical scenarios, and interactive self-assessment quizzes, are based on Love's personal journey, extensive research, and a genuine intention to assist fellow learners.

Throughout this book, you'll find practical tips, study strategies, and spiritually rooted encouragement to help you navigate this journey with confidence and grace. It serves as a reminder that beyond academic readiness, achieving success also involves nurturing a peaceful mindset, placing trust in God's guidance, and deriving strength from His assurances. As you engage with these pages, you will be reminded of the truth in *Isaiah 41:10*: "So do not fear, for I am with you; do not be dismayed, for I am your God. I will strengthen you and help you; I will uphold you with my righteous right hand." The assurance of God's presence and unwavering support can serve as the steadfast anchor you require at each stage, offering you strength, solace, and assurance as you navigate the demanding preparation journey.

Transitioning into an AGPCNP encompasses far more than mere knowledge acquisition; it entails accepting a divine calling, a sacred duty to offer healing, empathy, and optimism to those requiring assistance. The competencies you are honing will not only enable you to make a meaningful difference in people's lives through compassionate care but also to bring healing and hope to the ailing and vulnerable. As *Jeremiah 29:11* reminds us: "For I know the plans I have for you, declares the Lord, plans for welfare and not for evil, to give you a future and a hope." Know that this plan includes equipping you with everything you need to succeed, including faith, wisdom, and perseverance.

Furthermore, this book encourages you to view challenges not as roadblocks, but as opportunities for growth. When you face moments of doubt, let *Philippians 4:13* remind you: "I can do all things through Him who strengthens me." This verse is a powerful reminder that you are never walking this path alone—God is with you every step of the way, guiding you, empowering you, and helping you overcome every obstacle.

As you prepare for this exam, know that every hour of study, every prayer, and every step you take is a testament to your commitment to this noble profession. Your learned lessons, sacrifices, and faith will culminate in this moment of achievement. This book supports and uplifts your dedication, which reflects God's purpose for your life, on your journey.

Therefore, as you embark on this transformative journey to becoming an AGPCNP, remember to breathe deeply, approach this resource with an open heart, and immerse yourself fully to benefit from its supportive guidance. Trust in your preparation, capabilities, and the divine guidance for this calling. May your path be illuminated with a clear sense of purpose, fortified by unyielding determination, and enriched with a profound wellspring of faith.

With blessings and encouragement,

Love Christophers

INTRODUCTION: YOUR COMPREHENSIVE GUIDE TO AGPCNP EXAM SUCCESS

The journey to becoming a certified Adult-Gerontology Primary Care Nurse Practitioner (AGPCNP) is both exciting and challenging. Whether you're a recent graduate embarking on your first certification or a seasoned nurse practitioner seeking to validate your expertise, preparing for the AGPCNP exam can feel overwhelming. This book is here to change that.

In **preparing for the Adult-Gerontology Primary Care Nurse Practitioner (AGPCNP) Exam**, you'll find a step-by-step roadmap designed to simplify your preparation, boost your confidence, and ensure you're equipped with the tools and knowledge needed to excel.

Why This Book?

The AGPCNP exam isn't just a test of your knowledge; it's a measure of your ability to apply that knowledge in real-world clinical settings. Many candidates struggle not because they lack competence, but because they're unsure how to organize their preparation or apply test-taking strategies effectively. That's where this guide comes in.

This book offers:

- **A Structured Plan**: A detailed timeline to help you stay on track and avoid last-minute cramming.
- **High-Yield Content**: Clear, concise explanations of critical topics, from health promotion to chronic disease management.
- **Practical Examples**: Case studies and clinical scenarios that reflect the type of questions you'll encounter on the exam.
- **Test-Taking Strategies**: Proven techniques to tackle tricky questions, manage time effectively, and avoid common pitfalls.
- **Practice Questions**: Hundreds of questions with detailed rationales to solidify your understanding and improve your confidence.

Who Is This Book For?

This book is tailored to meet the needs of:

1. **Recent Graduates**: If you've just completed your nurse practitioner program, this guide will help you bridge the gap between coursework and certification.

2. **Experienced Practitioners**: For those re-entering the exam process after years in practice, this book offers a refresher on the latest evidence-based guidelines and standards.

3. **Working Professionals**: Balancing exam preparation with a busy schedule? This book's organized, efficient approach ensures you make the most of your study time.

What You'll Find in This Book

1. A Step-by-Step Study Plan

This book begins by helping you create a personalized study timeline. Whether you have two months or six months to prepare, you'll find guidance on allocating your time effectively.

Example:

In Week 1, focus on understanding screening guidelines and immunization schedules. Learn when to recommend a colonoscopy, mammogram, or bone density scan based on USPSTF recommendations.

2. High-Yield Topic Reviews

Each chapter dives into a critical area of the exam, breaking down complex concepts into manageable sections. Topics include:

- Health promotion and disease prevention.
- Pharmacological and non-pharmacological management.
- Advanced diagnostic reasoning.

- Chronic and acute disease management.

Example:
When reviewing pharmacology, you'll learn not only about first-line treatments for hypertension but also when to adjust therapy based on comorbidities such as diabetes or chronic kidney disease.

3. Case Studies and Clinical Scenarios

Real-world examples help you apply your knowledge in a clinical context. These scenarios mirror the questions you'll encounter on the exam.

Example:
A 70-year-old patient with Type 2 diabetes presents with leg pain and non-healing ulcers. How would you assess for peripheral arterial disease, and what is your first step in management?
This type of case prepares you to think critically and prioritize patient care.

4. Test-Taking Strategies

Learn how to navigate complex questions, eliminate incorrect answers, and prioritize patient safety. The book provides techniques tailored specifically to the AGPCNP exam format.

Example:
When faced with a "Select All That Apply" question, you'll learn to evaluate each option independently, avoiding the common pitfall of overthinking.

5. Practice Questions with Rationales

As they say, practice makes perfect. This book includes hundreds of questions designed to test your knowledge and improve your exam readiness. Detailed rationales explain why the correct answers are right—and why the incorrect ones are wrong.

Example:

A 65-year-old smoker presents for a routine check-up. What screening is recommended for lung cancer prevention?

- A) Chest X-ray
- B) CT scan
- C) Pulmonary function tests
- D) None
  Answer: **B** (low-dose CT scan for smokers aged 50-80 who meet specific criteria).

How to Use This Book

This book is more than just a study guide; it's your companion throughout the preparation process. Here's how to get the most out of it:

1. **Start with the Study Plan**: Use the suggested timeline to map out your preparation.
2. **Engage Actively**: Highlight key points, create flashcards, and summarize concepts in your own words.
3. **Practice Daily**: Dedicate time each day to answering practice questions and reviewing rationales.
4. **Simulate Exam Conditions**: Take full-length practice tests

to build stamina and confidence.

5. **Revisit Weak Areas**: Use the book's structure to focus on topics where you need improvement.

Why This Book Stands Out from Others on the Market

When it comes to preparing for the Adult-Gerontology Primary Care Nurse Practitioner (AGPCNP) exam, there's no shortage of resources available. So, what makes *Faith, Focus, and Fulfillment: Your Guide to Conquering the Adult-Gerontology Primary Care Nurse Practitioner (AGPCNP) Exam* with Grace different from the rest? This book is designed with your success in mind, blending practicality, clarity, and real-world application to give you an edge. Here's why this guide stands out from other options:

1. A Step-by-Step Approach

Many resources provide a wealth of information but lack a clear, actionable structure. This book offers a **step-by-step study plan** tailored to your timeline, whether you have two months or six to prepare. By breaking the preparation process into manageable sections, it ensures that you stay organized and focused.

Example:
Instead of overwhelming you with every possible exam topic at once, the book starts with foundational concepts like health promotion and builds to more complex subjects like pharmacology and care planning.

2. Real-World Clinical Scenarios

Unlike many exam guides that present dry, theoretical content, this book includes **real-world case studies and clinical scenarios** to help you apply what you've learned in a practical context. These scenarios mirror the questions you'll face on the exam and in your everyday practice as a nurse practitioner.

Example:

You'll encounter cases such as:

- *A 68-year-old male with a history of COPD presents with worsening shortness of breath. What diagnostic tests would you order, and how would you adjust his medication regimen?* These scenarios not only prepare you for the exam but also enhance your critical-thinking skills for clinical practice.

3. High-Yield, Exam-Focused Content

Some books overwhelm readers with extraneous details that are unlikely to appear on the exam. This guide focuses on **high-yield topics** that are most relevant to the AGPCNP exam, allowing you to maximize your study efficiency.

Example:

- Easy-to-understand summaries of the latest evidence-based guidelines, such as USPSTF screening recommendations and pharmacological protocols, ensure that you're studying what truly matters.

4. Detailed Practice Questions with Rationales

While many books include practice questions, this guide takes it a step further by offering **comprehensive rationales** for every answer. This ensures you not only understand the correct answer but also grasp why the other options are incorrect.

Example:

A 72-year-old female with osteoporosis is prescribed alendronate. What key instructions should you provide to ensure proper administration?

- A) Take with food to reduce gastrointestinal discomfort.
- B) Lie down immediately after taking the medication.
- C) Take with a full glass of water and remain upright for at least 30 minutes.
- D) Avoid calcium supplements while on this medication.

Correct Answer: C. The rationale explains the importance of remaining upright to prevent esophageal irritation, a common side effect of bisphosphonates.

5. Focus on Test-Taking Strategies

Many exam guides overlook the importance of **how** to take the test. This book dedicates a section to strategies that help you:

- Decode tricky questions.
- Manage your time effectively during the exam.
- Avoid common pitfalls like overthinking or second-guessing.

Example:

You'll learn how to approach "Select All That Apply" questions, such as evaluating each option independently to avoid confusion.

6. Comprehensive but Concise

While some books are overly dense, making it difficult to sift through the information, this guide is both **thorough and concise**. It delivers the depth you need without unnecessary complexity, helping you retain the material more effectively.

7. Evidence-Based and Up-to-date

The healthcare field evolves rapidly, and staying current is crucial. This book reflects the **latest evidence-based guidelines** and clinical best practices, ensuring that your preparation aligns with current standards.

Example:
It covers updated recommendations for managing chronic conditions like diabetes, hypertension, and COPD, as well as recent changes to USPSTF screening guidelines.

8. Built for All Learners

This book is designed to meet the needs of diverse learners by incorporating multiple learning methods:

- **Visual learners**: charts, diagrams, and tables simplify complex concepts.
- **Auditory learners**: Tips on integrating external resources like podcasts or audio courses.
- **Kinesthetic learners**: interactive exercises, such as creating SOAP notes and writing care plans.

9. Personalized Study Guidance

Unlike generic guides, this book helps you tailor your study plan based on your unique needs, strengths, and timeline. Whether you're balancing work, family, or other commitments, it offers strategies to help you integrate studying into your busy life.

10. Focus on Long-Term Success

While the immediate goal is passing the AGPCNP exam, this book is also a resource for your **ongoing career** as a nurse practitioner. It reinforces clinical reasoning and evidence-based practice, helping you transition from exam preparation to real-world application with confidence.

Example:

- Chapters on chronic disease management provide frameworks that you can use in your daily practice, not just for the test.

Final Thoughts

This book stands apart because it's more than just a study guide—it's a partner in your journey to becoming a certified AGPCNP. With its structured approach, real-world applications, and focus on both exam readiness and clinical success, it equips you with the tools you need to achieve your goals.

Whether you're preparing for your first certification or re-entering the field after years of practice, this guide is your trusted resource to help you succeed. Let this book be your roadmap, your mentor, and your confidence-builder as you take this important step in your professional journey.

CHAPTER 1
UNDERSTANDING THE AGPCNP EXAM

"The heart of the discerning acquires knowledge, for the ears of the wise seek it out."
Proverbs 18:15

Embarking on the journey to become a certified Adult-Gerontology Primary Care Nurse Practitioner (AGPCNP) is more than just a career decision—it is a calling. This role demands not only intellectual rigor but also resilience, compassion, and unwavering faith in your ability to make a difference. The AGPCNP exam is not just a test; it symbolizes the culmination of your commitment to mastering the art and science of caring for adults and elderly patients. It is a gateway to fulfilling your mission to serve with excellence, humility, and grace.

While preparing for this exam may seem daunting, with the right mindset, resources, and strategies, success is achievable. This chapter aims to equip you with a thorough comprehension of the exam's structure, content, and available resources. You'll discover not only what to expect but also how to navigate the preparation process with confidence and purpose.

The Importance of Understanding the Exam

This is what preparation feels like without first understanding the structure and requirements of the AGPCNP exam. Understanding the exam's format, content areas, and expectations helps you gain clarity and focus. This knowledge empowers you to:

- Identify key areas to concentrate your efforts.
- Avoid wasting time on irrelevant topics.
- Build confidence as you approach your study plan with intention.

As Proverbs 24:27 reminds us, "Prepare your work outside; get everything ready for yourself in the field, and after that build your house." Similarly, laying the groundwork for your preparation is the first step toward achieving your goal.

The Mission Behind the Exam

The AGPCNP exam is designed to assess your ability to provide holistic, evidence-based care for adults and older adults. It evaluates not only your knowledge of clinical guidelines and best practices but also your critical thinking, ethical decision-making, and capacity for patient-centered care. Passing this exam signifies your readiness to take on a role of profound responsibility and make a significant impact.

Consider this verse from Colossians 3:23: "Whatever you do, work heartily, as for the Lord and not for men." Your preparation for this exam is a reflection of your commitment to excellence in serving others.

What This Chapter Will Cover

This chapter will guide you through the following key aspects of understanding the AGPCNP exam:

1. **Exam Overview**: A high-level introduction to the exam's purpose and key content areas.

2. **Exam Certifying Bodies**: Insights into the differences between the ANCC and AANPCB exams.

3. **Exam Content Breakdown**: An in-depth look at the domains covered in each exam.

4. **Eligibility Requirements**: A checklist to ensure you meet the prerequisites for registration.

5. **Exam Format and Question Types**: A breakdown of the types of questions you'll encounter and how to approach them.

6. **Scoring and Passing Criteria**: What you need to know about achieving a passing score.

7. **Registration and Scheduling**: Practical tips for applying and choosing a testing location.

8. **Analyzing Strengths and Weaknesses**: Tools and techniques to assess your readiness.

9. **Developing a Study Timeline**: A step-by-step guide to creating a personalized study plan.

Each section is designed to provide actionable insights, practical examples, and a sense of empowerment to help you take charge of your preparation.

The Bigger Picture

Your decision to pursue AGPCNP certification is part of a larger story—one of growth, service, and transformation. As you begin this journey, remember that it's not just about passing an exam; it's about answering a higher calling to care for others with wisdom, skill, and compassion. Let this chapter serve as a compass, guiding you through the first steps of preparation with clarity and purpose.

"For I know the plans I have for you," declares the Lord, "plans to prosper you and not to harm you, plans to give you hope and a future." —Jeremiah 29:11

Let's dive in and take the first steps toward success together.

Exam Overview

The AGPCNP exam is not just a test of knowledge; it is a measure of your readiness to step into a role of profound responsibility—providing holistic, evidence-based care to adults and geriatric populations. This exam evaluates your ability to integrate clinical expertise with compassion and professionalism, ensuring the highest quality of care for your patients.

This journey calls for a steadfast commitment to your purpose. As 2 Timothy 2:15 reminds us, "Do your best to present yourself to

God as one approved, a worker who does not need to be ashamed and who correctly handles the word of truth." Approach this exam as an opportunity to demonstrate your dedication to excellence in nursing practice.

The AGPCNP exam evaluates your competence in four key areas:

1. Assessment

- The ability to gather and interpret critical patient information is foundational to the role of an AGPCNP. You will be evaluated on your ability to:
  - Collect thorough patient histories, including lifestyle factors, medical conditions, and family health.
  - Conduct comprehensive and focused physical exams.
  - Interpret diagnostic tests, such as lab results, imaging studies, and screenings, to formulate a clinical picture.

Example: You might encounter a case where a 65-year-old patient presents with fatigue and shortness of breath. You will need to assess their medical history for risk factors, auscultate for abnormal lung sounds indicative of respiratory conditions, and interpret lab results to discern underlying issues like anemia or cardiovascular abnormalities.

2. Diagnosis

- Recognizing patterns, differentiating among possible conditions, and pinpointing accurate diagnoses are critical skills. This domain evaluates:

  - Your ability to prioritize differential diagnoses.
  - Recognition of red-flag symptoms that require urgent attention.
  - Application of evidence-based criteria to confirm a diagnosis.

Example: A 72-year-old with Type 2 diabetes presents with a non-healing foot ulcer. The exam might ask you to differentiate between peripheral arterial disease and diabetic neuropathy based on clinical findings.

3. Treatment and Management

- A key aspect of a great AGPCNP is the ability to develop and implement individualized care plans, showcasing a commitment to personalized patient care. This section assesses your knowledge of:
  - Pharmacological interventions (e.g., appropriate medication selection, dosages, and monitoring).
  - Non-pharmacological strategies, such as lifestyle modifications, physical therapy, and counseling.
  - Chronic disease management, including conditions like hypertension, COPD, and diabetes.
  - Acute care for infections, injuries, or sudden exacerbations of chronic conditions.

Example: You may be asked to design a care plan for a patient with uncontrolled hypertension who is also managing chronic kidney disease. The correct answer would include first-line medications like ACE inhibitors, dietary adjustments, and regular monitoring of renal function.

4. Professional Role

- This domain focuses on the ethical and professional responsibilities of an AGPCNP, including:
  - Advocacy for patients, especially vulnerable populations.
  - Upholding ethical principles, such as autonomy, beneficence, and justice.
  - Incorporating evidence-based practice into patient care.
  - Understanding legal and regulatory aspects of practice, such as scope of practice and prescribing guidelines.

Example: A question might explore how you would advocate for a patient struggling to afford their medication by identifying resources like pharmaceutical assistance programs.

Certifying Bodies

The AGPCNP exam is offered by two certifying organizations:

- **American Nurses Credentialing Center (ANCC)**
  - Focuses on theory, clinical practice, and the professional

role of the nurse practitioner.

    - Includes advanced question formats like drag-and-drop, hot spot, and multiple-response questions.

- **American Academy of Nurse Practitioners Certification Board (AANPCB)**
    - Emphasizes clinically oriented questions that test diagnosis and management skills.
    - Primarily consists of multiple-choice, scenario-based questions.

Differentiating between these exams helps you choose the one that best matches your strengths and career objectives.

Key Resources

Preparation for the AGPCNP exam requires not only hard work but also the right tools. Here are some resources that combine theoretical knowledge, clinical application, and practice questions:

1. **ANCC Adult-Gerontology Primary Care Nurse Practitioner Review Manual**
    - Comprehensive and aligned with the ANCC exam blueprint.
    - Includes practice questions and case studies.
2. **Fitzgerald's Nurse Practitioner Certification Exam Prep**

  - Renowned for its detailed explanations and practical tips.
  - Provides clinical pearls and test-taking strategies.

3. **Leik Intensive Review**
   - High-yield content with concise summaries and practice exams.
   - Perfect for last-minute reviews and identifying weak areas.
4. **BoardVitals and AANP Prep (online practice tests)**
   - Offers customizable question banks and full-length practice exams.
   - Features rationales for correct and incorrect answers to deepen your understanding.

Inspiration for the Journey

As you prepare for the AGPCNP exam, remember Joshua 1:9: "Have I not commanded you? Be strong and courageous. Do not be afraid; do not be discouraged, for the Lord your God will be with you wherever you go."

Every hour you dedicate to preparation is an investment in your calling to heal and serve. Let this chapter and the tools within this book empower you to move forward with confidence, knowing that you are not alone in this journey.

Step 1: Understand the Exam

1. Exam Certifying Bodies

There are two organizations that offer the AGPCNP certification exam, each with its own distinct focus and format. Understanding the differences between these exams will help you choose the path that aligns with your strengths and career goals.

American Nurses Credentialing Center (ANCC)

- **Focus**: Combines theory, professional role, and clinical practice. The ANCC exam assesses your integration of advanced knowledge with ethical and professional responsibilities.
- **Exam Format**:
  - 175 questions (150 scored, 25 unscored pretest questions).
  - Includes multiple-choice, drag-and-drop, hot spot (click on image areas), and multiple response questions.
- **Time Limit**: 3.5 hours.
- **Cost**: $395 (discounted to $295 for ANA members).
- **Website**: ANCC AGPCNP Exam
- **Example**: You may encounter advanced question formats like identifying anatomical structures on an image or pri-

oritizing care steps in a clinical scenario. For instance, a drag-and-drop question might ask you to arrange the steps for managing a diabetic foot ulcer in the correct order.

American Academy of Nurse Practitioners Certification Board (AANPCB)

- **Focus**: clinically oriented, emphasizing diagnosis and management. The AANPCB exam evaluates your practical, real-world skills in providing daily patient care.
- **Exam Format**:
  - 150 questions (135 scored, 15 unscored pretest questions).
  - Multiple-choice, clinically based scenarios that reflect real-world practice.
- **Time Limit**: 3 hours.
- **Cost**: $315 (discounted to $240 for AANP members).
- **Website**: AANPCB AGNP Exam
- **Example**: Questions are often case-based, such as managing an elderly patient with COPD who presents with acute shortness of breath. You'll need to identify the most appropriate next steps in treatment.

Choosing the Right Exam

While both certifying bodies offer reputable credentials, your decision may hinge on considerations such as your career objectives, specialization interests, and preferred exam formats:

- If you prefer an exam that includes professional role responsibilities and theoretical concepts, the **ANCC** might be a better fit.
- If you're looking for a clinically focused exam with straightforward, case-based questions, the **AANPCB** may align better with your strengths.

Reflection: As you consider your options, keep Proverbs 3:6 in mind: "In all your ways acknowledge Him, and He will make your paths straight." Trust in your preparation and the direction you feel called to take.

2. Exam Content Breakdown

Both the ANCC and AANPCB exams evaluate your ability to assess, diagnose, and manage patients effectively. However, each exam has a slightly different emphasis, reflecting their unique focus areas.

1. **Assessment (35%)**: Focuses on your ability to collect and interpret patient information, including:
    - Taking thorough patient histories.
    - Conducting comprehensive physical exams.
    - Interpreting diagnostic tests such as lab results, imaging, and screenings.
2. **Diagnosis (25%)**: Tests your ability to formulate accurate

differential diagnoses and recognize disease patterns.

Example

: A 72-year-old with a non-healing leg ulcer may require you to differentiate between peripheral arterial disease and diabetic neuropathy.

3. **Plan (40%)**: Evaluates your knowledge of treatment options and care planning, including:
   - Selecting appropriate medications and dosages.
   - Implementing non-pharmacological strategies like dietary counseling or physical therapy.
   - Patient education, follow-up, and referrals.

ANCC Content Areas

1. **Assessment and Diagnosis (31%)**: Combines patient history-taking, physical exams, and diagnostic reasoning.

Example

: A question might involve identifying the next best step in evaluating a patient with abnormal lab findings, such as elevated liver enzymes.

2. **Plan of Care (38%)**: Focuses on your ability to:
   - Develop comprehensive treatment plans.
   - Manage chronic and acute conditions.
   - Implement evidence-based pharmacological and

non-pharmacological interventions.

3. **Professional Role (31%)**: Evaluates your understanding of ethics, patient advocacy, and evidence-based practice.

Example

: A scenario might explore how you would address an ethical dilemma, such as advocating for a patient who is refusing life-saving treatment due to cultural beliefs.

Action: Download the Test Blueprints

Blueprints are essential guides to understanding the scope and structure of the exams. Use them to prioritize your study efforts:

- AANP Exam Blueprint PDF
- ANCC Exam Blueprint PDF

Comprehending the content breakdown not only provides insight into the exam's structure but also enables you to tailor your study plan to match the exam's key areas, optimizing your preparation. Remember Proverbs 4:7: "The beginning of wisdom is this: Get wisdom. Though it cost all you have, get understanding." As you deepen your knowledge of the exam's content, you are equipping yourself to succeed and serve with excellence.

3. Exam Eligibility

Prior to registering for the AGPCNP exam, it is crucial to confirm that you satisfy all the eligibility criteria established by your selected certifying body. These criteria are designed to confirm that you have the foundational education, clinical experience, and licensure necessary to take on the responsibilities of an Adult-Gerontology Primary Care Nurse Practitioner.

Eligibility Requirements

1. **Educational Requirements**:
   - You must have earned a graduate degree (Master of Science in Nursing or Doctor of Nursing Practice) with a focus on Adult-Gerontology Primary Care.
2. **Clinical Hours**:
   - A minimum of 500 faculty-supervised clinical hours in an AGPCNP role is required.
3. **Licensure**:
   - You must hold an active and unencumbered Registered Nurse (RN) license in the state where you practice.

Practical Tip

Before submitting your application, verify your eligibility on the certifying body's website. Missing documentation or unmet requirements can delay your registration and testing timeline. Checklists and guidelines provided by the ANCC and AANPCB are invaluable for confirming your readiness.

- **ANCC Eligibility Information**: ANCC AGPCNP Exam Eligibility

- **AANPCB Eligibility Information**: AANPCB AGNP Exam Eligibility

By meeting these eligibility criteria, you demonstrate your commitment to the high standards expected of a nurse practitioner. As Psalm 90:17 reminds us, "Let the favor of the Lord our God be upon us, and establish the work of our hands upon us; yes, establish the work of our hands!" With diligence and preparation, you are laying the groundwork for a fulfilling and impactful career in advanced nursing practice.

4. Exam Format and Question Types

Comprehending the types of questions featured on the AGPCNP exam is vital for efficient preparation and optimal performance. The format varies slightly between the ANCC and AANPCB exams, but both are designed to test your clinical reasoning and application of knowledge.

Multiple-Choice Questions

- These questions present clinical scenarios and test your ability to recall, apply, and synthesize information. Each question typically has four options, with only one correct answer.

Example (AANP):

- *A 72-year-old patient with Type 2 diabetes presents with leg pain and non-healing ulcers. What is the most likely diagnosis?*
  - A) Peripheral arterial disease

- B) Neuropathy
- C) Deep vein thrombosis
- D) Cellulitis
- **Correct Answer**: A

Advanced Formats (ANCC-specific)

- The ANCC exam features advanced question types that demand interactive engagement and critical thinking:

1. **Hot Spot Questions**:
    - Identify specific areas on an image.
    - *Example*: You might be asked to click on the location of the mitral valve for auscultation on a chest diagram.
2. **Drag-and-Drop**:
    - Arrange items in the correct order based on a clinical process.
    - *Example*: Organize the steps for wound dressing or the sequence of actions in managing a patient with an asthma exacerbation.

These formats test not only your knowledge but also your ability to apply it in practical, real-world scenarios.

Understanding the exam's format will help you tailor your preparation and approach questions with confidence. Proverbs 19:20 reminds us, "Listen to advice and accept instruction, that you may gain wisdom in the future." With practice and focus, you can master these question types and succeed on exam day.

5. Scoring and Passing

Attaining a passing score on the AGPCNP exam remains your primary objective. Understanding the scoring criteria for both exams will help you set clear targets during your preparation.

AANP Scoring

- It requires a scaled score of at least **500 out of 800** to pass.
- The scoring system ensures fairness by adjusting for the relative difficulty of the questions.

ANCC Scoring

- Uses a scaled score of **350 out of 500** to pass.
- The scaled scoring accounts for varying difficulty levels across different exam versions.

Preparation Tip

- To ensure readiness, aim to consistently score **80–85%** on practice tests. This benchmark allows for a margin of error on the actual exam day.

Example: If you're scoring 85% on a 150-question practice test, you're answering approximately 128 questions correctly, well above the minimum passing threshold.

Final Encouragement: Remember the encouragement from Galatians 6:9 to persist in doing good, for in the right time, you will harvest the rewards if you do not lose heart. Each hour of study, each practice question, and each review session is an investment in your future as a compassionate and skilled nurse practitioner. With diligent preparation, success is within your reach.

6. Exam Registration and Scheduling

Registering for the AGPCNP exam is a straightforward process, but proper preparation ensures that you avoid delays and unnecessary stress. Here are the steps to follow:

Prepare Your Documents

To complete your application, you'll need to gather the following:

1. **Proof of Graduation**:
    - Submit a transcript or official letter verifying graduation from an accredited AGPCNP program.
2. **Clinical Hour Verification**:
    - Documentation confirming completion of the required 500 faculty-supervised clinical hours.
3. **Active RN License**:
    - Provide proof of your current and unencumbered RN

licensure.

Apply Online

Each certifying body operates through its own unique online application portal, necessitating a tailored approach for submitting your exam application. Select the appropriate link based on your chosen exam:

- **ANCC Application**: Apply Here
- **AANPCB Application**: Apply Here

Choose a Testing Location

Exams are administered at secure testing centers. You'll need to select a convenient location:

1. **ANCC**:
    - Administered through Prometric Testing Centers.
    - Locate a center: Prometric Testing Centers
2. **AANPCB**:
    - Administered through PSI Testing Centers.
    - Locate a center: PSI Testing Centers

Scheduling Your Exam

- Once your application is approved, you'll receive an Authorization to Test (ATT) email with instructions to schedule your exam.
- Book your test date early to secure your preferred time and location.

Final Encouragement: Proverbs 21:5 reminds us, "The plans of the diligent lead surely to abundance, but everyone who is hasty comes only to poverty." Taking the time to prepare your documents, apply early, and schedule wisely will set you on a path toward success. Careful planning can help you approach your exam with confidence and peace of mind.

7. Analyze Your Strengths and Weaknesses

Self-awareness is a crucial component of effective exam preparation. Identifying your strengths and areas for improvement allows you to allocate your study time strategically and maximize your readiness.

Self-Assessment Tools

1. **Diagnostic Pretests**:
    - Take a diagnostic test at the beginning of your preparation to pinpoint knowledge gaps.
    - Recommended tools:
        - BoardVitals Diagnostic Test
        - Fitzgerald Online Quizzes

2. **Track Your Progress**:
   - Use practice tests to monitor improvement over time.
   - Focus extra study time on weak areas while maintaining your strengths.

Tip

Allocate more time to content areas where you consistently score below your target threshold. For instance, if pharmacology is a weak point, dedicate additional hours to reviewing drug classes, indications, and contraindications.

8. Develop a Study Timeline

Creating a structured timeline keeps you on track and ensures comprehensive coverage of the material. Adjust the timeline based on your individual schedule and learning pace.

Suggested Timeline

1. **Total Study Time**:
   - Plan for **2-3 months** of preparation, depending on your familiarity with the content.
2. **Daily Commitment**:
   - Weekdays: **2-4 hours** per day.
   - Weekends: **4-6 hours** per day.

3. **Structured Weekly Plan**:

    - **Weeks 1-2**: Focus on health promotion and disease prevention.
    - **Weeks 3-4**: Dive into assessment and diagnosis.
    - **Weeks 5-6**: Concentrate on the plan of care, including pharmacological and non-pharmacological management.
    - **Weeks 7-8**: Conduct a full review of all topics and complete multiple practice tests.

Final Encouragement: Proverbs 21:5 reminds us, "The plans of the diligent lead surely to abundance, but everyone who is hasty comes only to poverty." Through meticulous evaluation of your strengths, improvement of your weaknesses, and adherence to a structured timeline, you are building a solid foundation for achieving success. Trust in your preparation and remain steadfast in your efforts. Victory is within reach.

As you prepare for the AGPCNP exam, remember the words of Isaiah 40:31: "But those who hope in the Lord will renew their strength. They will soar on wings like eagles; they will run and not grow weary; they will walk and not be faint."

Approach your preparation with diligence, faith, and confidence. This journey is not just about passing an exam; it's about stepping into your calling as a healer and advocate for your patients. Each hour spent studying is an investment in your ability to transform lives and provide compassionate, evidence-based care.

Let this book be your guide and companion every step of the way. Trust in your preparation, lean on your faith, and know that you are equipped to succeed in this noble calling. Remember, Philippians 4:13 declares, "I can do all things through Christ who strengthens me." You walk this path with unwavering support from your determination, your purpose, and the grace of God, guiding you through every step of this journey.

CHAPTER 2

DEVELOPING A STUDY PLAN

"Commit to the Lord whatever you do, and He will establish your plans."
Proverbs 16:3

Preparing for the AGPCNP (Adult-Gerontology Primary Care Nurse Practitioner) exam is a significant milestone in your professional journey. This exam not only tests your knowledge and skills but also serves as a gateway to advancing your career and making a meaningful impact on the lives of your patients. Success begins with imagining where you want to go and creating a clear plan to get there. Crafting a personalized study plan that aligns with your goals, schedule, and resources is essential to turning that vision into reality.

This chapter is your guide to creating a study plan that keeps you motivated, focused, and empowered. You will learn how to break down the exam preparation process into manageable steps, organize your time effectively, and use the right tools and resources to maximize your efforts. By following these steps, you will feel confident and determined as you approach the exam, boosting your confidence.

Success is not just about hard work—it's about working smart. A thoughtful study plan helps you prioritize what matters most, eliminates unnecessary stress, and builds your readiness step by step. Regardless of juggling a demanding job, family responsibilities, or other commitments, you will find in this chapter the strategies to stay on track and make steady progress. Keep in mind that this journey is about personal growth and persistence. Each small step you take brings you closer to reaching your goals.

Proverbs 16:3: "Commit your work to the Lord, and your plans will be established."

With faith, discipline, and determination, you can overcome challenges and turn your aspirations into accomplishments. Let's begin your journey to success by building a strong foundation—your personalized study plan.

Step 1: Set Your Exam Date

The first step in developing your study plan is setting a realistic exam date. This decision involves more than just selecting a day on the calendar; it involves establishing the foundation of your preparation. Choose a date that provides ample time to prepare—typically 3 to 6 months in advance. This timeframe ensures that you have sufficient time to master the content, practice test-taking strategies, and build the confidence you need to succeed.

Mark your chosen date boldly on your calendar. Let it serve as a visual reminder of your goal and a motivator to keep moving forward. Treat it as a commitment to yourself—a date that represents not just an exam but the culmination of your hard work and dedication.

Proverbs 21:5: "The plans of the diligent lead surely to abundance, but everyone who is hasty comes only to poverty."

Invest time in meticulous planning, recognizing that thorough preparation leads to abundance. Approach this decision with prayer and reflection to ensure that it aligns with your personal and professional commitments. Seek guidance to confirm that the timing is right and that you're setting yourself up for success.

Why 3 to 6 months?

- **Three Months**: This is ideal for those who already have a solid grasp of the core material and can dedicate more intensive daily study hours.

- **Six Months**: This extended period is better for those balancing work, family, or other responsibilities, as it allows for steady, consistent progress without feeling overwhelmed.

Example Timeline:

If you plan to take the exam in six months, divide your study period into manageable phases. Each phase will focus on specific content areas, ensuring comprehensive coverage. For instance:

- **Months 1-2**: Focus on health promotion and disease prevention.

- **Months 3-4**: Dive into pharmacology and system-specific content like cardiovascular and pulmonary disorders.

- **Months 5-6**: Concentrate on reviewing weak areas, taking practice tests, and refining test-taking strategies.

Consider Your Commitments:

Think about your current obligations, such as work, family, and personal activities. Acknowledge the time you can realistically dedicate to studying each week. For example:

- If you work full-time, aim for 2-3 hours on weekdays and 4-6 hours on weekends.

- If your schedule is more flexible, consider increasing your daily study hours to accelerate your preparation.

Practical Example:

Sarah, a full-time nurse practitioner, decided to take her AGPCNP exam in six months. She marked the exam date on her calendar and broke down her preparation into weekly milestones. By dedicating two hours each evening and four hours every Saturday, she was able to stay on track without sacrificing her work-life balance. Her consistent effort paid off when she passed the exam on her first attempt.

Key Takeaway:

Selecting your exam date is not just about setting a deadline; it's a commitment to your journey ahead. Be intentional, thoughtful, and prayerful as you make this decision. The date you choose will serve as the foundation of your study plan, directing each phase of your preparation.

Psalm 37:5: "Commit your way to the Lord; trust in Him, and He will act."

With a clear vision and a firm commitment, you are setting yourself on the path to success. Let this step serve as a declaration of your dedication and a reminder that with faith and preparation, you can achieve your goals.

Step 2: Establish a Study Timeline:

Setting a timeline is crucial, as it helps you structure your study plan effectively, prioritize tasks, and ensure comprehensive preparation.

An organized study schedule is your roadmap to success. It keeps you on track, reduces procrastination, and ensures that you thoroughly review all critical areas. Dedicate specific weeks to focusing on particular topics, and always prioritize consistency over intensity.

Week-by-Week Study Plan:

Weeks 1–2: Health Promotion & Disease Prevention

- **Focus**: Screenings, immunizations, lifestyle counseling, and prevention strategies.
- **Activities**:
  - Read relevant chapters in **Leik's Intensive Review** or **Fitzgerald's Review**.
  - Use flashcards or apps like **Quizlet** to memorize screening guidelines.
  - Complete practice questions on platforms like **BoardVitals** or **Pocket Prep**.
  - Watch video lectures or attend webinars on evidence-based health promotion techniques.
- **The goal is to** understand evidence-based guidelines and confidently apply them to case scenarios. To this end, students should create notes summarizing key concepts and revisit them weekly.

Weeks 3–4: Assessment & Diagnosis

- **Focus**: history-taking, physical exams, diagnostic tests, and differential diagnosis.
- **Activities**:
  - Study diagnostic reasoning using **Fitzgerald's Review** or **Barkley Certification Review**.
  - Practice interpreting lab results (e.g., CBC, lipid panel)

with resources like **Lab Tests Online**.

  - Use case studies to practice differential diagnosis and refine your clinical decision-making skills.
  - Take quizzes on patient presentations (e.g., fatigue, chest pain) to test your knowledge.

- **Goal**: Accurately assess and diagnose common conditions in primary care. Keep a journal to document challenging cases and revisit them regularly.

Weeks 5–6: Plan of Care

- **Focus**: Developing treatment plans, pharmacology, chronic disease management, and patient education.
- **Activities**:
  - Review pharmacology chapters in **Leik's Review** or attend a pharmacology webinar.
  - Create a chart for drug categories, side effects, and interactions. Use color-coded visuals for better retention.
  - Practice clinical scenarios focusing on chronic diseases like diabetes and hypertension.
  - Join a study group to discuss challenging pharmacological concepts.
- **The goal is to** formulate safe, effective, evidence-based care plans and develop cheat sheets summarizing drug classes and treatment protocols for quick reference.

Week 7: Comprehensive Review

- **Focus**: Reinforce weak areas, review notes, and complete practice tests.
- **Activities**:
    - Take a full-length timed practice test (e.g., from **AANP** or **ANCC**).
    - Review incorrect answers to address knowledge gaps. Use study guides to deepen your understanding of missed questions.
    - Revisit flashcards and charts for quick reinforcement.
    - Participate in mock study sessions with peers to test your readiness.
- **Goal**: Solidify knowledge and refine test-taking strategies. Use visualization techniques to imagine yourself succeeding on exam day.

Week 8: Final Preparation

- **Focus**: Test strategies, last-minute review, and mental readiness.
- **Activities**:
    - Review "Exam Tips" sections in study guides and focus on frequently tested topics.
    - Practice time management with shorter timed quizzes.
    - Ensure you have all required documents and know the

logistics for exam day.

    - Engage in relaxation techniques, such as deep breathing or mindfulness meditation, to reduce anxiety.

- **The goal is to** build confidence and reduce test anxiety. To ensure this, develop a pre-exam checklist to ensure you feel prepared and organized.

This schedule will guide you systematically through your AGPC-NP exam preparation, helping you balance your life's demands.

Step 3: Implement Diagnostic Resources:

Utilizing diagnostic tools is essential for identifying strengths and weaknesses, focusing study efforts efficiently, and tracking progress throughout the preparation process.

Harness the power of diagnostic tools to identify strengths and weaknesses. These tools will help you focus your energy on areas needing improvement and streamline your study efforts.

- **Pretests**: Start with a diagnostic pretest from **Fitzgerald**, **BoardVitals**, or **Leik's Review** to assess your baseline knowledge. These initial evaluations will help you understand where you stand and which areas require more focus.

- **Apps**: Use tools like **UWorld** and **Quizlet** for targeted practice. These apps provide interactive quizzes, flashcards, and detailed rationales to enhance understanding and retention.

- **Tracking Progress**: Keep a checklist of completed topics and areas needing review. Use digital tools like **Google Sheets**, **Notion**, or **Trello** to organize your progress visually. Color-coding tasks or setting reminders can help you stay on track.

2 Timothy 2:15: "Do your best to present yourself to God as one approved, a worker who has no need to be ashamed, rightly handling the word of truth."

By diligently monitoring your progress, you ensure that each step you take is meaningful and enhances your study sessions. Know that your effort is leading you closer to approval and accomplishment.

Step 4: Balance Study and Self-Care

Studying effectively requires more than time and effort; it demands a balance of physical, mental, and emotional well-being. Balancing your well-being will help you stay motivated and avoid burnout.

- **Take Breaks**: Follow the **Pomodoro Technique**—25 minutes of focused study followed by a 5-minute break. After every 4 cycles, take a longer 15-30 minute break to refresh your mind.

- **Stay Active.** Regular exercise reduces stress and boosts focus. Simple activities like walking, yoga, or light cardio can enhance mental clarity and energy levels.

- **Eat Well**: Maintain a balanced diet rich in whole foods, fruits, and vegetables to fuel your mind and body. Avoid excessive caffeine or sugary snacks that can lead to energy crashes.

- **Sleep**: Quality sleep is essential for enhancing memory and concentration. Aim for 7-9 hours per night, especially before practice tests and the actual exam.

Example:

When you feel overwhelmed, reduce your daily study hours while ensuring consistency. For instance, reduce study sessions to one hour per day and use the extra time for self-care activities like meditation or spending time with loved ones. This allows you to recharge and return with renewed energy and focus.

Philippians 4:6-7: "Do not be anxious about anything, but in every situation, by prayer and petition, with thanksgiving, present your requests to God. And the peace of God, which transcends all understanding, will guard your hearts and your minds in Christ Jesus."

Balancing study and self-care helps you approach your preparation with increased clarity and confidence. Remember, rest and rejuvenation are just as critical as the hours you dedicate to studying. Your mental and physical well-being are crucial assets in your path to success.

Step 5: Flexibly Adapt Your Plan:

Flexibility in adjusting your study plan is crucial to adapt to unforeseen circumstances, prioritize effectively, and optimize your preparation for success.

Life is unpredictable, and flexibility is key to maintaining progress. Adjusting your study plan doesn't mean failure—it means you're resilient and adaptable.

- **If you find yourself falling behind,** prioritize weak areas, streamline review of familiar topics, and utilize summary guides or videos to optimize time. Focus on high-weighted exam topics to maximize your efforts.

- **If Ahead**: Use extra time for additional practice tests or deeper dives into challenging subjects. Join study forums or attend live review sessions to gain fresh insights and perspectives.

Isaiah 40:31: "But they who wait for the Lord shall renew their strength; they shall mount up with wings like eagles; they shall run and not be weary; they shall walk and not faint."

Believe that you have the strength to adapt and persist when faced with challenges. Seek guidance and wisdom to navigate unexpected obstacles with steadfast determination. Being flexible in your approach will help you stay on track and maintain calmness and confidence during your preparation. Always remember that any progress, no matter how small, is meaningful and should be acknowledged.

Developing a study plan is not just about preparing for an exam; it's about growing into the confident, skilled practitioner you aspire to be. Every step you take—every chapter read, every quiz completed, every challenge overcome—is a testament to your dedication and resilience. Celebrate small achievements as you progress and always remember your ultimate goal.

Philippians 4:13: "I can do all things through Christ who strengthens me."

With determination, faith, and a well-crafted study plan, success is within your reach. Embrace the journey with confidence, knowing that each day of preparation brings you closer to your goals. You've got this!

CHAPTER 3

IMPORTANCE OF GATHERING RESOURCES FOR AGPNP EXAM PREPARATION

"The wise store up knowledge, but the mouth of a fool invites ruin."
Proverbs 10:14

Preparing for the AGPCNP (Adult-Gerontology Primary Care Nurse Practitioner) exam is a significant milestone in your journey as a nurse practitioner. The resources you choose can differentiate between feeling overwhelmed and stepping into the exam room with confidence. A well-chosen toolkit not only provides the knowledge you need but also helps you develop the skills and strategies required to succeed. This chapter explores why resources are vital and provides specific tips on how to select those that align with your unique learning style and needs, such as considering visual aids or audio lectures based on your preferred learning methods.

Tips for Selecting Resources

Having the right resources is essential for effectively preparing for the AGPCNP exam. These resources serve as the foundation for your success on the exam.

Success begins with careful planning and equipping yourself with the tools needed to master the content, ensuring that you approach the AGPCNP exam with confidence and readiness. Just as a craftsman needs the proper tools to create a masterpiece, you need well-selected study materials, tools, and platforms to excel. Each resource plays a vital role in building your knowledge, honing your skills, and boosting your confidence. This chapter will guide you through choosing and utilizing the best resources to support your journey. You will learn how to optimize your resource selection for effective exam preparation.

Taking the time to gather the right resources is a foundational step that ensures your preparation is efficient, organized, and comprehensive. For instance, Emily, an AGPCNP candidate, started her preparation by investing in a few key review books and joining a study group. She quickly realized that the shared insights from her peers, combined with high-quality materials, helped her grasp difficult concepts more easily. Similarly, Michael, who initially struggled with time management, found that using Trello to organize his tasks and

Google Calendar for scheduling study sessions allowed him to balance work, family, and exam preparation effectively. A well-prepared candidate is not only confident but also equipped to overcome challenges along the way. By learning from others' experiences and tailoring your approach to fit your unique needs, you can build a resource toolkit that works best for you.

Why Resources Matter

The AGPCNP exam covers a broad range of topics, from health promotion and pharmacology to differential diagnoses and chronic disease management. The right resources help you understand complex concepts through simplified explanations, stay updated on current evidence-based guidelines, practice and refine test-taking strategies, and develop confidence in applying theoretical knowledge to clinical scenarios.

- Understand complex concepts through simplified explanations.
- Stay updated on current evidence-based guidelines.
- Practice and refine test-taking strategies.
- Develop confidence in applying theoretical knowledge to clinical scenarios.

Investing time in selecting the best resources ensures that your study efforts are targeted and productive, saving you valuable time and reducing unnecessary stress during your preparation. For example, selecting a comprehensive review book like Fitzgerald's or Leik's can provide clear, structured content, helping you avoid the confusion of piecing together fragmented materials. Similarly, using apps like UWorld or Pocket Prep for on-the-go practice can streamline your preparation by allowing you to focus on weaker areas. By prioritizing tools that align with your learning style, such as visual aids or audio lectures, you can make your study time more efficient and engaging. Let's explore the categories of resources you'll need and how they can elevate your preparation.

The Power of Preparation

The foundation of success lies in thorough preparation. Before delving into the specifics of gathering resources, let's explore the significance of adequate preparation.

Imagine embarking on a journey without a map or compass. Gathering resources is like acquiring the navigation tools needed to chart your path to success. Resources provide direction, clarity, and a structured approach to your study process. Consider this step as the groundwork for everything you'll build in the coming months. By investing in high-quality materials, you set the stage for focused and efficient learning.

With the right resources in hand, you're equipped not only to pass the exam but to excel in your role as a nurse practitioner.

1. Books

Must-Have Review Books:

- **Leik's Adult-Gerontology Nurse Practitioner Certification Intensive Review** by Maria Codina Leik
    - Known for its concise summaries and high-yield content.
    - Includes two full-length practice exams and test-taking tips.
    - Ideal for quick reviews and last-minute prep.
    - **Example**: Sarah used Leik's book to create flashcards for pharmacology and found the practice questions invaluable for building confidence. She also used the practice exams to simulate real test conditions, which helped her manage exam anxiety.
    - *Available on Amazon*
- **Fitzgerald's Nurse Practitioner Certification Exam and Practice Preparation** by Margaret Fitzgerald
    - A comprehensive resource covering theory, clinical practice, and professional roles.
    - Includes tips for answering exam questions and detailed explanations of content areas.
    - Fitzgerald's approach integrates clinical reasoning with test strategies, making it a favorite among exam takers.
    - **Example**: Emily appreciated how Fitzgerald's book

broke down complex topics like differential diagnoses into manageable sections, helping her feel more confident in her clinical decision-making.

- *Available through Fitzgerald Health Education*

- **Adult-Gerontology Primary Care Nurse Practitioner Exam Secrets Study Guide** by Mometrix
  - Focuses on test-taking strategies alongside content review.
  - Includes practice questions with detailed rationales, which provide insight into common pitfalls and how to avoid them.
  - **Example**: Jason used this guide to develop a strategic approach to answering challenging exam questions, which significantly improved his practice test scores.
  - *Available on Mometrix*

Supplemental Books:

- **Pharmacology for the Primary Care Provider** by Marilyn Winterton Edmunds
  - A detailed pharmacology reference focusing on medications relevant to adult and geriatric populations.
  - Features real-world examples of medication use in primary care settings, making it a practical resource for clin-

ical scenarios.

   - **Example**: Maria used this book to deepen her understanding of drug interactions and side effects, which helped her tackle pharmacology questions with ease.
   - *Available on Elsevier*

- **Advanced Assessment: Interpreting Findings and Formulating Differential Diagnoses** by Mary Jo Goolsby and Laurie Grubbs
   - Ideal for honing diagnostic skills with case studies and diagnostic reasoning exercises.
   - Includes practical examples to bridge the gap between theory and clinical practice, making it a valuable tool for mastering assessment and diagnosis.
   - **Example**: David found the case studies in this book particularly helpful in preparing for the exam's scenario-based questions.

Books form the cornerstone of your study plan, providing in-depth insights, structure, and a wealth of information. Investing in these resources will help you build a strong foundation for success on the AGPCNP exam and beyond.

2. Online Courses

Online courses offer structured learning and expert guidance, providing in-depth coverage of AGPCNP exam content areas, interactive sessions, and strategies to enhance your test-taking skills and critical thinking abilities.
They're a great option for those who prefer interactive sessions and access to seasoned instructors. These courses not only cover exam content but also provide strategies to enhance your test-taking skills and critical thinking abilities.

Recommended Online Courses:

- **Fitzgerald Health Education Associates**
  - Offers live and on-demand certification review courses tailored to AGPCNP candidates.
  - Covers all AGPCNP exam content areas with depth and clarity, including health promotion, pharmacology, and disease management.
  - Includes downloadable materials, practice tests, and a Q&A section to address common concerns.
  - **Example**: Emily attended Fitzgerald's live course and found the interactive lectures and opportunities to ask questions invaluable. The downloadable materials allowed her to review key points on her own time.
  - *Available through Fitzgerald Health Education*
- **Barkley & Associates**
  - Provides comprehensive review courses with audio and

printed materials designed to simplify complex concepts.

- Includes online practice tests and pharmacology updates to ensure you're ready for current exam standards.
- **Example**: John used Barkley's course to strengthen his understanding of chronic disease management and pharmacological interventions. The printed study guides were especially helpful for quick reviews.
- *Available on Barkley & Associates*

- **BoardVitals**
  - Features customizable question banks and full-length practice exams tailored to the AGPCNP exam.
  - Offers progress tracking and performance analytics to pinpoint strengths and weaknesses, helping you focus your efforts effectively.
  - **Example**: Michelle used BoardVitals to simulate exam conditions and fine-tune her time management skills. The detailed explanations for each question improved her understanding of tricky concepts.
  - *Available on BoardVitals*

Why Choose Online Courses?

Online courses combine the expertise of seasoned instructors with the convenience of flexible scheduling. Whether you prefer live sessions for direct interaction or on-demand materials for self-paced learning, these courses adapt to your needs.

By harnessing the power of these courses, you acquire insights from experts, adhere to a structured learning path, and cultivate the confidence to excel in your AGPCNP exam preparation. They represent an investment not only in exam success but also in your development as a skilled and capable nurse practitioner.

3. Practice Tests

Practice tests are indispensable for gauging your readiness and fine-tuning your test-taking strategies. They simulate real exam conditions and help identify areas that need improvement. Regular practice not only boosts your confidence but also ensures you are familiar with the exam format, time constraints, and question styles.

Recommended Practice Tests:

- **ANCC Practice Test**:
    - Official practice tests for the ANCC AGPCNP exam.
    - Designed to simulate real exam conditions with a focus on clinical reasoning and evidence-based decision-making.
    - **Example**: Amanda used the ANCC practice tests to get accustomed to the format and pacing of the actual exam,

which helped reduce her anxiety on test day.

- *Available through ANCC Practice Tests*

- **AANPCB Practice Test**:
  - Offers sample questions specifically tailored to the AANPCB exam.
  - Includes clinical scenarios and management questions, making it an excellent resource for primary care-focused preparation.
  - **Example**: David found these tests instrumental in building his critical thinking skills, as they closely mirrored real-life patient care scenarios.
  - *Available through AANPCB Practice Tests*
- **Exam Edge**:
  - Provides a variety of practice tests for the AGNP exam with customizable options for difficulty and length.
  - Includes detailed explanations for both correct and incorrect answers, fostering a deeper understanding of the material.
  - **Example**: Sophia used Exam Edge to build her stamina for full-length tests and improve her time management. The detailed rationales helped her identify and address weak areas.
  - *Available on Exam Edge*

Benefits of Practice Tests:

1. **Simulate Exam Conditions**: Familiarize yourself with the format, question style, and time constraints of the actual exam.
2. **Identify Weaknesses**: Highlight areas that require further study, allowing you to focus your efforts where they matter most.
3. **Build Confidence**: Repeated exposure to exam-style questions reduces test anxiety and improves readiness.
4. **Enhance Test-Taking Skills**: Develop strategies for managing tricky questions, pacing yourself, and making educated guesses when needed.

Integrating regular practice tests into your study routine enhances your skills, enriches your understanding, and prepares you for exam day with confidence and certainty.

4. Mobile Apps

Mobile apps are perfect for studying on the go. They offer bite-sized content, interactive features, and the flexibility to learn anytime, anywhere. With features like detailed rationales, performance tracking, and daily quizzes, mobile apps enhance your study experience by pro-

viding personalized and engaging learning opportunities.
Whether you're commuting, taking a lunch break, or waiting in line, mobile apps make it easy to reinforce your knowledge and practice exam concepts.

Recommended Mobile Apps:

- **Pocket Prep**
    - Offers AGNP-specific practice questions with detailed rationales to deepen understanding.
    - Features daily quizzes and performance tracking to keep you motivated and on track.
    - **Example**: Sarah used Pocket Prep to tackle daily quizzes during her breaks, which helped her identify and improve weak areas incrementally.
- **UWorld**
    - Renowned for high-quality question banks and in-depth rationales that focus on clinical reasoning and test-taking strategies.
    - User-friendly interface allows for seamless navigation between questions and explanations.
    - **Example**: Carlos used UWorld during his lunch breaks to review high-yield questions and rationales, which enhanced his critical thinking skills.
- **Quizlet**

- Create or access flashcards for topics like pharmacology, diagnostic criteria, and screening guidelines.
- Offers a collaborative platform where users can share and access pre-made study sets.
- **Example**: Emily used Quizlet to create custom flashcards for pharmacology and shared them with her study group, making collaborative learning both fun and effective.

Benefits of Mobile Apps:

1. **Convenience**: Study anytime, anywhere, turning idle moments into productive learning opportunities.
2. **Customization**: Tailor your learning experience with personalized flashcards, quizzes, and topic-specific practice.
3. **Engagement**: Interactive features and bite-sized content make studying more enjoyable and less overwhelming.

By incorporating mobile apps into your study plan, you can make consistent progress, stay motivated, and maximize your preparation time efficiently.

5. Websites and Guidelines

Staying updated with evidence-based guidelines is crucial for the AG-PCNP exam and clinical practice, ensuring that your knowledge aligns with current standards of care and best practices.
Guidelines and trusted websites provide authoritative information that enhances both your exam preparation and your ability to deliver high-quality patient care.

Key Websites and Guidelines:

- **CDC Immunization Guidelines**: CDC Immunization Schedules
    - Regularly updated schedules and best practices for immunizations.
    - **Example**: Amanda reviewed the CDC's latest immunization schedules to ensure her knowledge on vaccine timing and eligibility was up to date.
- **USPSTF Screening Guidelines**: USPSTF Recommendations
    - Evidence-based recommendations for preventive services.
    - **Example**: Jason relied on USPSTF guidelines to refine his understanding of age-appropriate screenings and preventive measures for various populations.
- **American Diabetes Association (ADA)**: ADA Standards of Care
    - Comprehensive guidance on managing diabetes in di-

verse populations.

- **Example**: Maria used ADA standards to reinforce her approach to managing patients with Type 2 diabetes during case-based practice scenarios.

- **American Heart Association (AHA)**: AHA Guidelines
  - Authoritative resources on cardiovascular care, including hypertension and heart failure management.
  - **Example**: David referred to AHA guidelines for evidence-based recommendations on cardiovascular disease prevention.

Benefits of Using Guidelines:

1. **Accuracy**: Trusted guidelines ensure your knowledge is aligned with current standards of care.
2. **Comprehensiveness**: Cover a wide range of clinical topics essential for both exam preparation and practice.
3. **Relevance**: Help you prepare for questions based on real-world scenarios.

6. Study Groups and Forums

Collaboration can enhance your preparation by offering fresh perspectives, shared resources, and mutual encouragement. Connecting with a community of like-minded individuals enables you to acquire insights, discover new strategies, and maintain motivation throughout your study path.

Recommended Platforms:

- **Facebook Groups**:
  - **"AGNP Certification Study Group"**: A space to connect with peers preparing for the AGPCNP exam. Members share resources, ask questions, and offer support.
  - **"NP Students and New Grads"**: A supportive group for new nurse practitioners, offering tips for exam preparation and early career advice.
  - **Example**: Sarah joined the "AGNP Certification Study Group" and discovered a wealth of shared resources, including practice test recommendations and flashcards created by other members. The group also provided encouragement during challenging weeks.
- **AllNurses Forum**:
  - Features dedicated discussion boards for NP exam preparation and career guidance.
  - Includes threads where users share their study plans, discuss challenging topics, and celebrate milestones like

passing the exam.

- **Example**: Maria joined the AllNurses forum and gained valuable advice from experienced NPs, including tips for tackling pharmacology questions and staying focused during long study sessions.

Benefits of study Groups and Forums:

1. **Shared Resources**: Members often share study guides, notes, and links to helpful tools and materials.
2. **Motivation**: Engaging with others can help keep you accountable and inspired to stay on track with your study plan.
3. **Problem Solving**: Discussing difficult topics with peers can provide clarity and new perspectives, helping you overcome roadblocks in your preparation.
4. **Networking: Establishing connections with fellow candidates and practicing NPs can provide access to mentorship and professional opportunities.**

Tips for Effective Collaboration:

- Set clear goals for your participation in groups, such as finding specific resources or clarifying challenging concepts.
- Be an active participant by asking questions, sharing insights, and offering support to others.

- Use the group's collective wisdom to refine your study plan, but remain discerning about the accuracy and relevance of shared resources.

Engaging with study groups and forums not only enhances your learning experience but also reminds you that you are not alone in this journey. Together, you and your peers can achieve success, supporting one another every step of the way.

7. Audio Resources

Audio resources are excellent for passive learning during commutes, workouts, or while multitasking. They provide an opportunity to reinforce knowledge and gain insights without requiring dedicated screen time, making them a flexible and practical addition to your study routine.

Recommended Audio Resources:

- **Fitzgerald Audio Review**:
    - High-quality audio lectures covering exam content comprehensively.
    - **Example**: Emily listened to Fitzgerald's audio lectures during her morning commute, which helped her retain key concepts in pharmacology and health promotion.

- **Barkley Audio Series**:
    - Includes recordings of lectures and clinical scenarios that bring theoretical knowledge to life.
    - **Example**: David found the case-based discussions in the Barkley Audio Series particularly helpful for understanding diagnostic reasoning and treatment plans.
- **Podcasts**:
    - **The NPTE Clinical Files Podcast**: Offers case-based learning with real-world examples, making it ideal for honing critical thinking skills.
    - **Nurse Practitioner Podcast**: Provides updates on NP practice, certification tips, and practical advice for new and experienced NPs alike.
    - **Example**: Maria enjoyed listening to podcasts during her evening walks, finding them both engaging and informative.

Benefits of Audio Resources:

1. **Convenience**: Learn on the go without the need for a screen or textbook.
2. **Reinforcement**: revisiting key topics in a different format strengthens retention.
3. **Engagement**: Dynamic discussions and scenarios make

complex concepts easier to understand.

Tips for Using Audio Resources:

- Incorporate audio learning into your daily routine, such as during commutes or household tasks.
- Take notes on key points or follow along with supplemental materials when possible.
- Revisit particularly challenging topics multiple times to ensure comprehension.

Audio resources allow you to make the most of your time, turning everyday moments into opportunities for growth and learning.

8. Tools for Study Organization

Keeping your preparation organized is key to staying on track and avoiding overwhelm. The right tools for study organization can help you manage your time effectively, prioritize tasks, and visualize progress, ensuring a streamlined and stress-free preparation process.

Recommended Tools:

- **Notion or Trello**:

  - Digital study planners that allow you to track progress, set goals, and organize materials.
  - Use templates to log topics covered, schedule study sessions, and track practice test scores.
  - **Example**: Jane used Trello to create a visual board where she categorized study tasks as "To Do," "In Progress," and "Completed." This helped her stay motivated and on top of her goals.

- **Google Calendar**:
  - Schedule study sessions and set reminders for deadlines to maintain consistency.
  - Color-code events by topics or tasks to easily track your schedule.
  - **Example**: Michael set daily reminders for study blocks and weekly goals using Google Calendar, ensuring he stayed on track without overcommitting.

- **Mind Mapping Tools**:
  - Visualize key concepts and relationships between topics with tools like XMind or MindMeister.
  - Ideal for complex subjects like pharmacology or differential diagnoses.
  - **Example**: Linda used mind maps to link pharmacological treatments with common diagnoses, reinforcing her understanding of clinical connections and making it

easier to recall during practice tests.

Benefits of Study Organization Tools:

1. **Clarity**: Break down large tasks into manageable steps, reducing overwhelm.
2. **Accountability**: Track progress and celebrate milestones, keeping yourself motivated.
3. **Efficiency**: Spend less time figuring out what to study and more time focused on learning.
4. **Flexibility**: Easily adjust your plan as needed, ensuring you stay on track even when life happens.

Tips for Effective Organization:

- Dedicate time each week to review your study schedule and adjust based on progress.
- Use "time-blocking" to allocate specific hours to different topics or activities.
- Integrate reminders and checklists to ensure no task is overlooked.

Through effective use of organizational tools, you can turn your preparation into a structured and purposeful path, maximizing your efforts and reaching your goals with confidence.

By using organizational tools, you can transform your preparation process into a structured and focused journey, ensuring that you maximize your efforts and achieve your goals with confidence.

By gathering these resources, you'll establish a strong toolkit for AGPCNP exam preparation, setting the foundation for success in your journey as a nurse practitioner. Remember, the quality of your resources directly impacts your readiness and confidence, so choose wisely to ensure you are well-prepared for the AGPCNP exam. Select tools that match your learning style, and believe that with commitment and faith, you can achieve your objective.

CHAPTER 4

MASTERING CORE CONTENT

"Do your best to present yourself to God as one approved, a worker who does not need to be ashamed and who correctly handles the word of truth."
2 Timothy 2:15

Preparing for the AGPCNP exam requires more than just memorizing facts; it demands a profound understanding of the core concepts that define primary care practice. This chapter focuses on common conditions you are likely to encounter, such as hypertension, diabetes mellitus, and depression. Mastering these topics not only ensures exam readiness but also enhances your ability to deliver high-quality, evidence-based care to your patients.

These foundational conditions represent the backbone of primary care and are intricately linked to many of the questions you will face on the exam. Delve deeply into guidelines, case studies, and clinical reasoning to equip yourself with the tools for success in both test scenarios and real-world practice.

This chapter provides practical strategies, illustrative examples, and thought-provoking case studies to enhance your understanding of key concepts.

As you navigate this chapter, remember that your commitment to understanding these core areas reflects your dedication to becoming a proficient and compassionate nurse practitioner. Let's explore how to approach these topics systematically, integrate them into your study routine, and apply them with confidence.

Importance of Understanding Common Conditions for Exam Success and Clinical Practice

Understanding and mastering common conditions is essential not only for passing the AGPCNP exam but also for your role as a skilled primary care provider. Each of these conditions represents a cornerstone of clinical practice, requiring a comprehensive understanding of guidelines, clinical decision-making, and patient-centered care. Below, we'll explore hypertension, diabetes mellitus, and depression, offering actionable insights, case studies, and examples to enhance your preparation and clinical acumen.

Hypertension

Hypertension is one of the most prevalent chronic conditions encountered in primary care. Managing it effectively requires familiarity with evidence-based guidelines and the ability to individualize care for diverse patient populations.

- **Review JNC-8 Guidelines**:
    - **First-line treatments**:
        - ACE inhibitors (e.g., lisinopril)
        - ARBs (e.g., losartan)
        - Calcium channel blockers (e.g., amlodipine)
        - Thiazide diuretics (e.g., hydrochlorothiazide)
    - **BP targets**:
        - <140/90 mmHg for most adults.
        - <130/80 mmHg for patients with diabetes or chronic kidney disease.

- **Example Question**:
    - A 58-year-old male with diabetes and hypertension is on lisinopril but has uncontrolled BP (156/94 mmHg). What would be the next step?

- Add a calcium channel blocker or thiazide diuretic to his regimen for uncontrolled BP (156/94 mmHg).

Diabetes Mellitus

Diabetes mellitus is a complex chronic condition with significant implications for morbidity and mortality. A thorough understanding of the ADA Standards of Care is critical for effective management.

- **Study ADA Standards of Care**:
    - **Glycemic targets**:
        - HbA1c < 7% for most non-pregnant adults.
        - Individualize targets based on patient age, comorbidities, and risk of hypoglycemia.
    - **First-line treatment**:
        - Metformin remains the gold standard for Type 2 Diabetes management.
    - **Lifestyle modifications**:
        - Emphasize dietary changes, physical activity, and weight loss as key components of care.
- **Case Study**:

- **Subjective**: A 65-year-old male reports fatigue and polyuria.
- **Objective**: HbA1c of 9.5%, BMI of 32.
- **Plan**:
    - Initiate metformin 500 mg daily with gradual titration.
    - Provide dietary counseling, including the benefits of a Mediterranean diet.
    - Encourage 30 minutes of moderate exercise, 5 days a week.
    - Schedule follow-up in 3 months to reassess HbA1c and adherence.

Depression

Depression is a common mental health condition that significantly impacts quality of life. Recognizing its symptoms and initiating appropriate treatment is a vital aspect of primary care.

- **Familiarize with DSM-5 Criteria**:
    - Symptoms include:
        - Depressed mood.
        - Loss of interest or pleasure in activities.
        - Fatigue, changes in appetite, insomnia or hypersom-

nia, and feelings of worthlessness.

- Symptoms must persist for at least 2 weeks.

◦ **First-line treatment**:

- SSRIs (e.g., sertraline, fluoxetine) are the mainstay of pharmacological therapy.

- **Example Question**:

◦ A 72-year-old female presents with fatigue and weight loss. What labs and screenings are priorities?

- Order a TSH, CBC, and PHQ-9 for lab and screening priorities: TSH for hypothyroidism, CBC for anemia, and PHQ-9 for depression assessment.

By mastering these common conditions, you'll excel in the AG-PCNP exam and build a solid foundation for delivering exceptional patient care. Use these guidelines, case studies, and questions as a roadmap for success, ensuring you're well-prepared for both the exam and real-world clinical scenarios.

Strategies for Enhancing Study Efficiency and Knowledge Application

Effective studying is not about how much time you spend but how well you utilize it. Here are practical strategies to optimize retention and application of knowledge:

1. Organize Your Study Sessions

- **Proverbs 24:27**: "Prepare your work outside; get everything ready for yourself in the field, and after that build your house." Setting up a study-friendly environment lays the foundation for productive sessions.**Create a Dedicated Study Space**: creating a dedicated study space is crucial for maintaining focus and productivity during study sessions. Ensure your study area is well-lit, comfortable, and free from distractions to optimize your learning environment.
  - Choose a quiet, clutter-free environment that promotes focus and minimizes distractions.
  - Keep essential study materials within reach, such as textbooks, notebooks, highlighters, pens, and any reference materials relevant to your study topics.
  - Use tools like noise-canceling headphones or white noise apps if needed to enhance concentration.
- **Set Daily Goals**:
  - Break topics into manageable chunks to avoid feeling overwhelmed.
  - **Example Daily Plan**:
    - **Morning**: Study hypertension management and re-

lated guidelines.

- **Afternoon**: Complete 50 practice questions on hypertension.
- **Evening**: Review mistakes, analyze rationales, and summarize key points.

- **Use Time Management Techniques**:
    - **Utilize the Pomodoro Technique** by working intensely for 25 minutes followed by a 5-minute break. After completing four cycles, take a longer break of 15-30 minutes to recharge. This structured approach helps maintain focus and prevent burnout during study sessions.
    - **Time Blocking**: Implement time blocking by assigning specific time slots for various study tasks. For example, allocate 9:00-10:30 AM for reading materials and 2:00-3:30 PM for practicing exam questions. This structured approach helps you focus on different study activities effectively.

2. Begin with Challenging Topics: Strengthening Areas of Difficulty First

- **2 Corinthians 12:9**: "My grace is sufficient for you, for my power is made perfect in weakness." Focusing on weak areas helps transform vulnerabilities into strengths, empowering you for success.**Prioritize Topics**:

    - Focus on areas identified as weak during your diagnostic pretest or initial self-assessment.
    - Spend more time on challenging subjects such as pharmacology, geriatrics, or differential diagnosis to build a strong foundation in these critical areas.
    - **Leik's Intensive Review**: Offers concise explanations and high-yield summaries for targeted review.
    - **Fitzgerald Health Modules**: enroll in topic-specific modules to deepen your understanding of challenging subjects.
    - **Barkley & Associates**: leverage detailed lectures and practice questions to reinforce difficult concepts.
- **Recommended Study Resources for Strengthening Weak Areas:**
- **Example Approach**:
    - If pharmacology is a weak area:
        - Allocate 2-3 study sessions per week to review drug classes, mechanisms, and side effects.
        - Create flashcards for high-yield medications and practice applying them in clinical scenarios.

By starting with weak areas, you can build confidence and ensure that no gaps remain in your preparation, ultimately strengthening your overall readiness for the AGPCNP exam.

3. Use Active Learning Techniques,

Active Learning Techniques: Enhancing Knowledge Retention and Application

Active learning engages your brain more effectively than passive reading, helping you retain and apply knowledge. Here are strategies to make your study sessions dynamic and impactful:

- **Note-Taking**:
  - Summarize key points in your own words to enhance understanding and retention.
  - Use the Cornell Notes method to organize information:
    - Divide your page into three sections: main notes, cues/questions, and a summary at the bottom.
    - Write key concepts in the main section, jot questions or prompts in the cues section, and summarize your learning at the end.
- **Flashcards**:
  - Create physical or digital flashcards using apps like Quizlet for quick reviews.
  - **Example**:
    - **Front**: What is the first-line treatment for hypertension in diabetics?

        - **Back**: ACE inhibitors or ARBs (per ADA guidelines).

- **Diagrams and Charts**:
    - Visualize information by creating diagrams, charts, or mind maps to illustrate relationships between concepts.
    - **Tools**: Use platforms like XMind or MindMeister for digital mind mapping.
    - **Example**: Create a flowchart showing the progression of hypertension management based on JNC-8 guidelines.
- **Practice Scenarios**:
    - Apply knowledge by writing SOAP (Subjective, Objective, Assessment, Plan) notes for hypothetical patients.
    - **Example**:
        - Subjective: A 55-year-old male presents with fatigue and weight loss.
        - **Objective**: Elevated glucose, BMI 30.
        - **Assessment**: Likely Type 2 Diabetes Mellitus.
        - **Plan**: Lifestyle counseling, start metformin, follow-up in 1 month.

Incorporating active learning techniques into your study routine not only makes studying more engaging but also equips you with the skills to apply your knowledge effectively in clinical practice and on the exam.

4. Daily Practice Questions for Mastery: Reinforcing Knowledge and Test-Taking Skills Daily

Practice questions are invaluable for reinforcing knowledge, identifying weak areas, and building confidence in your test-taking abilities. Incorporating them into your daily study routine will ensure steady progress.

- **Set a Question Goal**:
  - Start with a manageable goal, such as 50-100 questions per day.
  - Gradually increase the number as you build stamina to simulate full-length exams.
- **Resources**:
  - **BoardVitals**: Offers customizable question banks with detailed rationales.
  - **Pocket Prep**: Provides quick quizzes and performance tracking for on-the-go study sessions.
- **Analyze Each Question**:
  - Review the rationales for both correct and incorrect answers to deepen your understanding.

- Identify patterns in your mistakes to target specific areas for improvement. For example, if you frequently misinterpret lab values, dedicate additional time to studying lab diagnostics.

- **Simulate Test Conditions**:
  - Schedule weekly timed practice tests to mimic the real exam environment.
  - Use official practice exams from ANCC or AANPCB to familiarize yourself with the format and question styles.

Incorporating daily practice questions not only reinforces what you've learned but also ensures you're prepared to tackle the exam with precision and poise.

5. Engage in Peer Learning

Collaboration with peers can provide new perspectives, shared resources, and mutual encouragement. Peer learning not only reinforces your understanding but also fosters a sense of camaraderie during your exam preparation journey.

- **Join Study Groups**:
  - Collaborate with others to discuss challenging topics and share insights.
  - Exchange notes and explain concepts to one anoth-

er—teaching is a powerful way to solidify your own knowledge.

- **Example**: Sarah joined a local study group where members took turns presenting on complex topics like pharmacology and differential diagnosis, which helped her grasp difficult material more effectively.

- **Participate in Online Forums**:
  - Join platforms like AllNurses or Facebook groups specifically for AGNP candidates.
  - Ask questions, share strategies, and celebrate milestones together.
  - **Example**: John found a supportive Facebook group where he received advice on managing test anxiety and discovered useful resources like practice exams and flashcards.

By collaborating with peers, you can broaden your understanding, gain new insights, and stay motivated throughout your study process.

6. Review Regularly

Regular review is essential for long-term retention and mastery of exam content. Spaced repetition and weekly recaps are two powerful strategies to ensure material stays fresh in your memory.

- **Proverbs 10:14**: "The wise lay up knowledge, but the mouth of a fool brings ruin near." Spaced repetition helps build wisdom steadily over time through reinforced learni ng.**Spaced Repetition**:
    - Review material at increasing intervals to solidify retention.
    - **Example**:
        - **Day 1**: Learn a new topic (e.g., pharmacology basics).
        - **Day 3**: Conduct a brief review of the material.
        - **Day 7**: Focus on reinforcing weak areas and practicing related questions.
    - Dedicate one day each week to reviewing all material covered during the week.
    - Use a combination of notes, flashcards, and practice questions to reinforce knowledge.
    - **Example**: On Sundays, spend two hours revisiting material covered during the week, focusing on weak areas and reattempting challenging practice questions.
- **Weekly Recaps**:

7. Focus on Test-Taking Strategies

Mastering test-taking strategies is as important as understanding the content. These techniques can help you approach the exam with confidence and improve your performance.

- **Eliminate Wrong Answers**:
  - Rule out distractors to narrow down your choices.
  - Look for keywords like "most likely," "first action," or "priority," which often guide you to the correct answer.
- **Prioritize Patient Safety**:
  - Always choose answers that address safety and immediate needs in clinical scenarios.
  - For example, when faced with a question about a patient experiencing chest pain, prioritize actions such as administering oxygen or obtaining an EKG.
- **Time Management**:
  - Divide your time evenly across sections to avoid rushing through questions.
  - Skip challenging questions initially and return to them later to maximize efficiency.

By focusing on these strategies, you can optimize your performance, manage stress, and confidently navigate the exam environment.

8. Reinforce Key Topics

Mastering test-taking strategies is as important as understanding the content. These techniques can help you approach the exam with confidence and improve your performance.

- **Eliminate Wrong Answers**:
    - Rule out distractors to narrow down your choices.
    - Look for keywords like "most likely," "first action," or "priority," which often guide you to the correct answer.
- **Prioritize Patient Safety**:
    - Always choose answers that address safety and immediate needs in clinical scenarios.
    - For example, when faced with a question about a patient experiencing chest pain, prioritize actions such as administering oxygen or obtaining an EKG.
- **Time Management**:
    - Divide your time evenly across sections to avoid rushing through questions.
    - Skip challenging questions initially and return to them later to maximize efficiency.

By focusing on these strategies, you can optimize your performance, manage stress, and confidently navigate the exam environment.

9. Stay Motivated

Maintaining motivation throughout your study journey is essential for sustaining focus and achieving your goals. Here are strategies to keep your energy and determination high:

- **Example**: Emily rewarded herself with a relaxing evening out after finishing a particularly difficult pharmacology review module.**Track Progress**:
    - Use a checklist or app to mark completed topics, giving you a clear sense of accomplishment.
    - Celebrate milestones, such as completing 1,000 practice questions or mastering a challenging subject.
    - Keep reminders of why you're pursuing certification, such as a photo of a patient who inspired you or a note with your career goals.
    - Write motivational quotes or affirmations in your study space to inspire perseverance.
    - Plan small rewards for achieving daily or weekly study goals, such as enjoying a favorite snack, watching a

movie, or taking a relaxing walk.

- Use larger rewards to celebrate significant accomplishments, like completing a full-length practice test or finishing a study module.

- **Example**: Sarah placed a note on her desk that read, "I will pass this exam and provide exceptional care to my patients. "**Visualize Success**:

- **Committing your work to the Lord and aligning your plans with your purpose can lead to success by ensuring that your efforts are driven by a meaningful goal.Rew ard Yourself**:

By tracking your progress, visualizing your goals, and rewarding yourself along the way, you'll stay motivated and energized, making your exam preparation journey both effective and fulfilling.

Reinforcing key topics ensures that you have a solid grasp of essential knowledge areas critical for the AGPCNP exam. Here's how to effectively solidify your understanding:

- **Pharmacology**:
  - Memorize drug classes, indications, side effects, and contraindications.
  - Use mnemonics to simplify complex information.
  - **Example**: "ABCD for Hypertension Management"
    - **A**: ACE inhibitors/ARBs.
    - **B**: Beta blockers.

        - **C**: Calcium channel blockers.
        - **D**: Diuretics.
    - **Psalm 119:66**: "Teach me good judgment and knowledge, for I believe in your commandments." Understanding pharmacology is crucial for making sound clinical decisions.
- **Screening and Guidelines**:
    - Familiarize yourself with USPSTF guidelines and updates.
    - **Example**: Mammograms for average-risk women start at age 50, every 2 years.
- **Proverbs 4:13**: "Keep hold of instruction; do not let go; guard her, for she is your life." Reinforcing key topics is your lifeline to exam success and clinical competence.**Chronic Disease Management**:
    - Study evidence-based approaches for managing conditions like diabetes, hypertension, COPD, and heart failure.
    - Use case studies and clinical scenarios to apply guidelines to patient care.
- **Eliminate Wrong Answers**:
    - Rule out distractors to narrow down your choices.
    - Look for keywords like "most likely," "first action," or

"priority," which often guide you to the correct answer.

- **Prioritize Patient Safety**:
  - Always choose answers that address safety and immediate needs in clinical scenarios.
  - For example, when faced with a question about a patient experiencing chest pain, prioritize actions such as administering oxygen or obtaining an EKG.
- **Time Management**:
  - Divide your time evenly across sections to avoid rushing through questions.
  - Skip challenging questions initially and return to them later to maximize efficiency.

By focusing on these strategies, you can optimize your performance, manage stress, and confidently navigate the exam environment.

10. Combine Study and Self-Care

Balancing study efforts with self-care is essential for maintaining focus, reducing stress, and achieving optimal performance. Here's how to integrate self-care into your study routine:

- **Sleep**:

    - Aim for 7-8 hours of quality sleep each night to enhance memory consolidation and cognitive function.
    - Create a consistent bedtime routine to signal your body it's time to rest.

- **Exercise**:
    - Stay active by incorporating regular physical activity into your day, such as walking, yoga, or light cardio.
    - Exercise reduces stress, boosts energy, and improves mental clarity, helping you approach study sessions with focus.

- **Breaks**:
    - Take short breaks during study sessions to refresh your mind. Use techniques like the Pomodoro Method to structure these breaks effectively.
    - Engage in relaxing activities during breaks, such as stretching, meditating, or listening to calming music.

By combining study with intentional self-care practices, you'll sustain your energy, maintain a positive mindset, and prepare yourself not only for the AGPCNP exam but also for the demands of your future career.Maintaining motivation throughout your study journey is essential for sustaining focus and achieving your goals. Here are strategies to keep your energy and determination high:

- **Example**: Sarah placed a note on her desk that read, "I will pass this exam and provide exceptional care to my patients. "**Visualize Success**:
    - Keep reminders of why you're pursuing certification, such as a photo of a patient who inspired you or a note with your career goals.
    - Write motivational quotes or affirmations in your study space to inspire perseverance.
- By tracking your progress, visualizing your goals, and rewarding yourself along the way, you'll stay motivated and energized, making your exam preparation journey both effective and fulfilling.
- Plan small rewards for achieving daily or weekly study goals, such as enjoying a favorite snack, watching a movie, or taking a relaxing walk.
- Use larger rewards to celebrate significant accomplishments, like completing a full-length practice test or finishing a study module.

Reinforcing key topics ensures that you have a solid grasp of essential knowledge areas critical for the AGPCNP exam. Here's how to effectively solidify your understanding:

- **Pharmacology**:
    - Memorize drug classes, indications, side effects, and contraindications.

- Use mnemonics to simplify complex information.
- **Example**: "ABCD for Hypertension Management"
    - **A**: ACE inhibitors/ARBs.
    - **B**: Beta blockers.
    - **C**: Calcium channel blockers.
    - **D**: Diuretics.
- **Psalm 119:66**: “Teach me good judgment and knowledge, for I believe in your commandments.” Understanding pharmacology is crucial for making sound clinical decisions.

- **Screening and Guidelines**:
    - Familiarize yourself with USPSTF guidelines and updates.
    - **Example**: Mammograms for average-risk women start at age 50, every 2 years.
- **Proverbs 4:13**: “Keep hold of instruction; do not let go; guard her, for she is your life.” Reinforcing key topics is your lifeline to exam success and clinical competence.**Chronic Disease Management**:
    - Study evidence-based approaches for managing conditions like diabetes, hypertension, COPD, and heart failure.

    - Use case studies and clinical scenarios to apply guidelines to patient care.

- **Eliminate Wrong Answers**:
    - Rule out distractors to narrow down your choices.
    - Look for keywords like "most likely," "first action," or "priority," which often guide you to the correct answer.
- **Prioritize Patient Safety**:
    - Always choose answers that address safety and immediate needs in clinical scenarios.
    - For example, when faced with a question about a patient experiencing chest pain, prioritize actions such as administering oxygen or obtaining an EKG.
- **Time Management**:
    - Divide your time evenly across sections to avoid rushing through questions.
    - Skip challenging questions initially and return to them later to maximize efficiency.

By focusing on these strategies, you can optimize your performance, manage stress, and confidently navigate the exam environment.

Mastering core content and implementing these effective study strategies will empower you to approach the AGPCNP exam confidently and prepared. Remember, preparation is not just about passing a test—it's about becoming the knowledgeable and compassionate nurse practitioner you aspire to be.

CHAPTER 5

TEST-TAKING STRATEGIES

"The plans of the diligent lead to profit as surely as haste leads to poverty."
Proverbs 21:5

Success on the AGPCNP exam isn't just about what you know; it's about how effectively you can apply that knowledge under pressure. Effective test-taking strategies can boost your confidence and performance. This chapter provides actionable tips, and empowering techniques to help you excel.

Step 1: Elimination Method

Elimination is a highly effective method for addressing multiple-choice questions. By narrowing down answer choices, you increase your chances of choosing the correct response. This method not only saves time but also boosts your confidence in tackling questions, especially when you're uncertain about the right answer.

- **Identify Clearly Incorrect Answers:**
    - Cross out options that are factually wrong, irrelevant to the scenario, or contradictory to established guidelines.
    - Focus on what remains to make an informed choice, ensuring you're leveraging your clinical knowledge and reasoning.
- **Identify Distracting Options:**
    - Test writers often include distractors that seem plausible but don't align with evidence-based practices. Be cautious of answers that:
        - Are overly broad or extreme (e.g., "always" or "never").
        - Are outside the scope of practice for an AGPCNP.
        - Contradict clinical guidelines or safety protocols.
- **Example**:
    - **Question**: A 65-year-old smoker presents for a routine check-up. What is the recommended preventive screening?
        - **A)** Colonoscopy

- **B)** Chest X-ray
- **C)** Low-dose CT scan
- **D)** PSA test

  - **Answer**: **C** (Low-dose CT scan is recommended for lung cancer screening in smokers aged 50-80). In this scenario:
    - Colonoscopy (A) is unrelated to smoking history.
    - Chest X-ray (B) is not the standard for lung cancer screening.
    - PSA test (D) is specific to prostate cancer, not relevant to smoking.

- **Tip**: After eliminating distractors, focus on the remaining options and compare them to the question's key details to make an informed choice. If you're left with two plausible choices, prioritize the option that ensures patient safety or aligns most closely with guidelines.
- **Practice Application**:
  - Incorporate this method into practice tests. For each question, consciously identify and eliminate incorrect answers before making your final selection.

Practical Time Management Scenario: Imagine you have 30 minutes left in the exam with 10 questions remaining. Allocate about 3 minutes per question to ensure you address each one effectively while still allowing time for a final review.

Efficient time management ensures that you have adequate time to address all questions without feeling rushed. It is not just about answering questions quickly but about managing your focus and energy to sustain optimal performance throughout the exam.

- **Tip**: Familiarize yourself with the exam's timing during practice tests to develop a comfortable rhythm.**Understand the Time Allotment**:
    - **For the ANCC exam,** you have 3.5 hours to answer 175 questions, which gives you around 72 seconds per question.
    - **AANPCB**: 3 hours for 150 questions (approximately 72 seconds per question).
- **Divide Your Time**:
    - Allocate between 1 to 1.2 minutes for each question to stay on track.
    - Allocate the remaining time for reviewing flagged questions or double-checking your answers.
    - **Example Strategy**:

- If the exam is divided into sections, calculate how many questions you need to complete per hour to stay within the time limit.

- **Example**: A pharmacology question with complex drug interactions feels overwhelming. Flag it, select a likely answer, and revisit it if time permits. **Flag Challenging Questions**:
  - For challenging questions, guess, flag, and proceed to the next.
  - Return to flagged questions during your review time.
- **Save Time for Review**:
  - Reserve the last **10-15 minutes** for a comprehensive review of flagged questions.
  - Focus on ensuring calculations, clinical guidelines, and rationale align with the question requirements.
- **Ephesians 5:15-16**: "Look carefully then how you walk, not as unwise but as wise, making the best use of the time." Remember, effective time management reflects wisdom and preparation.**Maintain Composure During Stress:**
  - If you find yourself falling behind, don't panic. Speed up slightly, but focus on maintaining accuracy.

Practical Example

Imagine you're taking the AANPCB exam. You start with a clinical scenario requiring you to prioritize care for a patient with multiple chronic conditions. The question is lengthy and time-consuming:

Scenario: A 60-year-old female presents with uncontrolled hypertension, Type 2 diabetes, and complaints of chest pain. What is your immediate priority?

- If you know the answer, proceed confidently. If unsure, eliminate obviously incorrect answers, make your best guess, and flag the question for review.
- By moving on quickly, you prevent yourself from losing valuable time for other questions.

Final Tip

During practice sessions, use a stopwatch to time how long you take for each question. Reflect on whether you're spending too long on certain topics, and adjust your pacing as needed. Consistent practice will make time management second nature.

Step 3: Practice Regularly

Recommended Practice Test Resources: Consider utilizing platforms like Fitzgerald Review, BoardVitals, and Pocket Prep for comprehensive practice questions covering a wide range of topics.

Practice tests are invaluable for building confidence, identifying weak areas, and refining strategies. Regular practice helps you become familiar with the exam's format, question types, and time constraints. It's through consistent effort and repetition that you solidify knowledge and boost your readiness.

- **Example**: Schedule Monday and Tuesday for pharmacology, Wednesday for cardiovascular topics, and Thursday for diabetes management. Use Fridays to review mistakes from the week.**Set Weekly Goals**:
    - Commit to completing **200+ practice questions** each week. Breaking this into smaller daily goals—like 30 questions a day—makes it manageable and ensures steady progress.
    - Focus on covering a range of topics, ensuring you don't neglect areas of weakness.
- **Resources**:
    - **Fitzgerald Review**: Offers practice quizzes after each chapter to reinforce key concepts.
    - **BoardVitals**: Provides customizable question banks and detailed rationales to help you understand why an answer is correct or incorrect.
    - **Pocket Prep**: Perfect for on-the-go quick quizzes, allowing you to make use of spare moments.
- **Example**: Allocate a Saturday morning for a 3-hour simulated test session. Treat it as a dress rehearsal for exam day.**S imulate Exam Conditions**:
    - Take full-length, timed practice tests in a quiet, distraction-free environment. Use the same time allotment as the actual exam to build endurance and test-day stamina.

- Avoid pausing or checking notes during these tests to mimic real exam conditions.

- **Example**: If you frequently miss pharmacology questions about drug interactions, dedicate extra time to studying drug classes and side effects using flashcards or charts.**Analyze Performance**:
    - Carefully review rationales for both correct and incorrect answers. This helps identify patterns in your mistakes, such as misinterpreting keywords or skipping steps in clinical reasoning.
    - Keep a journal of frequently missed questions or concepts to revisit them later.
- **Incorporate Spaced Repetition**:
    - Revisit previously studied topics at increasing intervals to enhance long-term retention. Tools like Anki or Quizlet's spaced repetition feature can help.

Step 4: Understand Question Types

-tical Tips for Recognizing Question Types: Engage in ques- -anks that offer diverse formats such as multiple-choice, -drop, and clinical scenario questions to sharpen your ability and respond to different question structures.

Familiarity with question formats reduces surprises and boosts confidence. Knowing what to expect allows you to focus on applying your knowledge effectively. Understanding the types of questions you will encounter can help you feel prepared and in control.

- **Multiple-Choice Questions (MCQs)**:
  - The most common format used by both ANCC and AANPCB exams.
  - Each question presents a scenario and 4-5 answer options, with only one correct choice.
  - **Tip**: Focus on the key details in the scenario to determine the best answer. Eliminate options that are factually incorrect or irrelevant.
- **Advanced Formats (ANCC Only)**:
  - **Drag-and-Drop**:
    - Requires arranging items in a specific sequence (e.g., steps in a diagnostic process).
    - **Example**: arrange the steps for conducting a head-to-toe physical assessment.
  - **Hot Spot**:
    - Involves clicking on a specific area of an image t identify a location (e.g., auscultation points for l sounds).
  - **Multiple Responses**:

        - You must select all correct answers (e.g., symptoms of a condition).
        - **Tip**: Carefully read the question stem to ensure you select all applicable choices.

- **Clinical Scenario Questions**:
    - These questions assess your ability to evaluate patient cases, apply clinical guidelines, and make decisions regarding care.
    - Often test advanced critical thinking and prioritization skills.
    - **Example**:
        - **Scenario**: A 72-year-old female with Type 2 diabetes presents with increased thirst and frequent urination. Her A1C is 9.5%. What is the best next step?
        - **Answer**: Initiate metformin and counsel on lifestyle changes. This reflects evidence-based practice for managing newly diagnosed Type 2 diabetes with elevated A1C.

Why Familiarity Matters

- **Reduce Test Anxiety**: Knowing the types of questions you'll face prevents surprises and helps you focus on answering effectively.

- **Boost Efficiency**: Understanding the structure of each question type allows you to approach them strategically.
- **Enhance Clinical Decision-Making**: Many question formats simulate real-life scenarios, helping you connect knowledge to practice.

Practical Tips for Success

1. **Practice Advanced Formats**:
    - Use resources like ANCC practice tests to familiarize yourself with drag-and-drop and hot spot questions.
    - Review visual aids in study materials to prepare for image-based questions.
2. **Focus on Clinical Scenarios**:
    - Study case studies that reflect common conditions and guidelines. Practice writing SOAP notes to reinforce decision-making skills.
3. **Utilize High-Quality Question Banks**:
    - Resources like BoardVitals and Fitzgerald Review offer question banks that mirror the complexity of real exam questions.
4. **Reinforce Foundational Knowledge**:
    - Strong knowledge of pharmacology, diagnostics, and clinical guidelines will make it easier to navigate any

question format.

Step 5: Apply Strategic Approaches

Practical Tips for Recognizing Question Types: Engage in question banks that offer diverse formats such as multiple-choice, drag-and-drop, and clinical scenario questions to sharpen your ability to identify and respond to different question structures.

Strategic approaches are essential for answering questions efficiently and accurately, especially in high-pressure exam settings. By honing your ability to interpret and prioritize questions, you'll improve both confidence and performance.

- **Focus on Keywords**:
  - Pay close attention to directive words like **first action**, **most likely**, **best**, or **priority**. These words provide vital clues about what the question is asking.
  - **Example**: If a question asks, "What is the first action for a patient presenting with chest pain?" focus on interventions that address immediate safety and stabilization.
- **Rule Out Distractors**:
  - Eliminate answers that are factually incorrect, unsafe, or irrelevant to the scenario.
  - Be cautious of options that sound plausible but contra-

dict clinical guidelines or evidence-based practices.

- **Tip**: If two answers seem correct, choose the one that prioritizes patient safety or aligns most closely with clinical standards.

- **Trust Your Instincts**:
  - Your first choice is often correct. Avoid second-guessing unless you identify a clear mistake in your reasoning.
  - **Example**: For a question about managing a patient with suspected sepsis, prioritize interventions that address fluid resuscitation and antibiotics rather than secondary assessments.
- **Apply Clinical Prioritization Frameworks**:
  - Use established frameworks like **ABCs (Airway, Breathing, Circulation)** to prioritize actions in emergency scenarios.
  - **Example**: A patient with respiratory distress should have their airway addressed before any other interventions.
- **Practice Scenarios**:
  - **Imagine a scenario where a 55-year-old male arrives with shortness of breath and cyanosis. What would be your initial step?**
    - **A)** Administer albuterol inhaler.
    - **B)** Start oxygen therapy at 2L/min.

   - **C)** Perform a full physical assessment.
   - **D)** Obtain a detailed history of symptoms.
   - **Answer**: **B** (Start oxygen therapy). Addressing airway and breathing takes precedence over other actions.

- **Analyze Each Question Thoroughly**:
   - Break down complex scenarios into manageable components:
      i. Identify the key issue.
      ii. Focus on the patient's immediate needs.
      iii. Apply evidence-based guidelines to select the best answer.

Step 6: Prioritize Safety and Guidelines

Mnemonic Devices for Guideline Recall: Create memory aids like 'ABCD for Hypertension Management' to remember key drug classes and their indications, aiding in quick recall during exam scenarios.

Many questions test your ability to prioritize patient safety and apply clinical guidelines. A clear understanding of these principles allows you to make decisions that reflect best practices and ensure the highest standard of care for your patients.

- **Patient Safety**:
  - Always prioritize actions that address immediate needs, such as **airway, breathing, and circulation (ABCs)**.
  - Consider the consequences of delaying an intervention, especially in critical scenarios.
  - **Example**:
    - **Scenario**: A patient with acute shortness of breath is cyanotic and unable to speak in full sentences.
      - The correct first step: Ensure the airway is clear and initiate oxygen therapy. Actions like obtaining a history or performing a physical exam should come after stabilization.
  - **Tip**: When in doubt, choose the answer that ensures patient safety and prevents harm.
- **Guidelines**:
  - Familiarity with evidence-based guidelines is essential for answering questions accurately. Use them as a foundation for clinical decision-making.
  - **Screening Recommendations**:
    - **Mammograms**: Begin at age 40 for average-risk women every 2 years and continue through age 74 **(USPSTF)**. Begin at age 40 for average-risk women

every 2 years and continue through age 74. The American Cancer Society (ACS) recommends that women between 40 and 44 have the option to start screening with a mammogram every year.

- **Colonoscopies**: Every 10 years, starting at age 45 for average-risk adults.
- **Bone Density**: Women aged 65+ or younger women with significant fracture risk should undergo DEXA scans.

- **Pharmacology Principles**:
  - **Hypertension in Diabetics**: ACE inhibitors or ARBs are the first-line treatment to protect kidney function.
  - **Hyperlipidemia**: Statins are indicated for patients with diabetes or cardiovascular risk factors.
  - **Tip**: Use mnemonics to remember key drug classes and their indications (e.g., "ABCD for Hypertension Management"—ACE" inhibitors, Beta blockers, Calcium channel blockers, Diuretics).
- **Chronic Disease Management**:
  - **Diabetes**:
    - A1C goal: <7% for most patients.
    - First-line therapy: Metformin, alongside lifestyle modifications.

- **Example**: A 60-year-old patient with an A1C of 8.5% and obesity. The best intervention: Start metformin, counsel on diet and exercise, and schedule a follow-up.

Step 7: Manage Exam Anxiety

Overcoming Anxiety Story: Consider sharing a narrative of a nursing student who successfully managed exam anxiety through mindfulness techniques and positive affirmations, showcasing the power of mental preparation.

Anxiety can impact performance, so it's crucial to prepare mentally and emotionally. Managing exam anxiety involves building resilience, focusing on the moment, and leveraging strategies that enhance your emotional well-being.

- **Practice Mindfulness**:
  - Use breathing exercises to calm your mind and body. Try the **4-7-8 breathing technique**: inhale for 4 seconds, hold your breath for 7 seconds, and exhale for 8 seconds.
  - Incorporate visualization techniques by imagining yourself confidently answering questions and achieving success.
  - Consider short meditation sessions or mindfulness apps like Headspace or Calm to build mental clarity.

- **Stay Positive**:
    - Focus on one question at a time. Avoid overanalyzing previous answers or worrying about the next question.
    - Replace negative thoughts with empowering affirmations such as, "I have prepared thoroughly, and I can handle this challenge."
    - Remember, every question is an opportunity to demonstrate your knowledge.
- **Example**: Before starting a practice test, visualize the exam environment. As you take the test, focus on steady breathing and treat each question as a fresh challenge.**Take Breaks**:
    - If the exam allows, take brief breaks to reset your focus. Use this time to stretch, breathe, or hydrate.
    - Use these moments to pray or center yourself, reminding yourself of your hard work and preparation.
- **Prepare Your Mind and Body**:
    - Get plenty of sleep the night before your exam to ensure mental clarity.
    - Avoid over-caffeinating, as it can exacerbate feelings of anxiety.
    - Eat a balanced meal before the test to maintain energy levels.
- **Remember Your Faith**:

  - **Philippians 4:13**: "I can do all things through Christ who strengthens me."Lean on scripture and prayer to fortify your confidence. Reflect on verses that inspire strength and courage, such as:

- **Example of Overcoming Anxiety**:
  - Sarah, a nurse practitioner student, found herself overwhelmed before her certification exam. By practicing deep breathing and focusing on one question at a time, she turned her nerves into determination. Her mantra, "I've prepared for this moment," helped her maintain focus and pass with outstanding results.

By managing anxiety effectively, you create an environment where your preparation and knowledge can shine. Trust in your hard work, lean on your faith, and approach the exam with resilience and confidence.

Step 8: Review Answers

Double-Check Numerical Consistency: Before submitting your exam, ensure that numerical answers, such as medication dosages, are in the correct units and align with the question requirements to prevent calculation errors.

Before submitting your exam, it is essential to review your flagged questions to ensure accuracy and completeness. This step helps you catch errors, clarify uncertainties, and maximize your score.

- **Example**: You flagged a question about the first-line treatment for heart failure. On revisiting, confirm the guideline-based answer and ensure you didn't misinterpret the question stem.**Reassess Flagged Questions**:

- Return to flagged questions with a calm and fresh perspective. Often, stepping away from a question briefly allows you to see it more clearly.
- Avoid overthinking or changing answers unless you identify a clear error or overlooked detail.
- **Tip**: Trust your preparation and instincts. Many candidates second-guess themselves unnecessarily, leading to errors.

- **Example**: A dosage calculation requires converting kilograms to pounds. Double-check that you applied the correct conversion factor and administered the appropriate dose. **Double-Check Critical Data**:
  - Verify all calculations, lab values, and dosages to ensure accuracy.
  - Ensure that numerical answers, such as medication dosages, match the units and requirements stated in the question.
  - Confirm that your selected answer aligns with the patient scenario and clinical guidelines provided in the question stem.
- **Review Rationales in Practice Tests**:
  - Use practice exams to develop a habit of revisiting flagged questions and analyzing both correct and incor-

rect answers. This will strengthen your ability to evaluate flagged items during the real exam.

- **Stay Focused on High-Yield Topics**:
    - Pay extra attention to questions related to frequently tested subjects like pharmacology, chronic disease management, and diagnostic interpretation.
    - **For instance,** if a patient has high glucose levels, make sure your answer follows the correct treatment order, such as starting with lifestyle changes and then considering metformin.

Step 9: Avoid Common Pitfalls

Maintaining Focus and Pacing Tip: Keep a steady pace during the exam to address all questions while monitoring the time. Avoid spending too long on individual questions to ensure you cover all sections effectively.

While navigating through the exam, being mindful of common pitfalls can save time and improve accuracy. Awareness and preparation are your best defenses against these traps.

- **Overthinking**:
    - Stick to the scope of the question and avoid adding assumptions or irrelevant details. Trust the information

provided and base your answer on it alone.

- **Tip**: Remember, questions are designed to test your knowledge, not to trick you. Focus on clarity and relevance.
- **Example**: For a question asking about the most likely diagnosis for fatigue and weight loss, rely on the given lab values and patient history instead of speculating about unmentioned factors.

- **Changing Answers**:
    - Avoid second-guessing unless you can clearly identify a mistake in your initial response.
    - Research shows that your first instinct is often correct.
    - **Example**: If you answered that an ACE inhibitor is the first-line treatment for hypertension in diabetics, resist the urge to change it unless the question explicitly disqualifies that choice.
- **Example**: If you have 3 hours to complete 150 questions, aim to finish each set of 50 questions in 1 hour, leaving at least 15 minutes for flagged items.**Ignoring Time**:
    - Keep a consistent pace and monitor the clock to ensure all questions are addressed. Use your flagged questions as a guide for review time.
    - **Tip**: Divide your time evenly across sections and leave a buffer for review at the end.

By mastering these test-taking strategies and practicing consistently, you'll enter the exam room with confidence and readiness. Remember, this journey is about more than passing a test—it's about becoming the competent, compassionate nurse practitioner you are meant to be. Trust that every challenge you've faced has prepared you for this moment.

You are prepared, capable, and supported every step of the way. Go forth with faith, resilience, and determination—you've got this!

By mastering these test-taking strategies and practicing consistently, you'll enter the exam room with confidence and readiness. Remember, this journey is about more than passing a test—it's about becoming the competent, compassionate nurse practitioner you are meant to be.

CHAPTER 6
NURTURE YOUR RELATIONSHIPS

"A friend loves at all times,
and a brother is born for a
time of adversity."
Proverbs 17:17

Being a caregiver often requires you to immerse yourself in your responsibilities to the point where your personal relationships become secondary. The constant demands on your time, energy, and emotions may limit meaningful interactions with your loved ones. These connections are essential for sustaining your spirit, providing vital support, and bringing joy.

The truth is, no one was designed to carry life's burdens alone. Ecclesiastes 4:9-10 beautifully reminds us, "Two are better than one because they have a good return for their labor. If either of them falls down, one can help the other up." This wisdom highlights the power of partnerships and the importance of leaning on others in times of need. Whether it's a spouse, a trusted friend, or a close family member, nurturing your relationships ensures that you have companions who can lift you up when the weight of caregiving becomes too much to bear.

Supportive relationships not only lend a listening ear but also offer solace during uncertainties, celebrate your victories, and extend a helping hand precisely when you require it most. These bonds are not built overnight; they require intention, time, and care to grow. When nurtured, they become a source of strength that empowers you to keep going, even in the face of life's challenges.

In this chapter, we will discuss ways to strengthen and care for your relationships while managing the challenges of caregiving. You'll learn practical strategies to maintain strong connections, foster deeper bonds, and create a network of love and encouragement. By investing time in nurturing these relationships, you enhance your own life and strengthen your capacity to be a compassionate and resilient caregiver.

Ecclesiastes 4:9-10: "Two are better than one because they have a good return for their labor: If either of them falls down, one can help the other up."

1. Stay Connected with Friends and Family: This section discusses the significance of maintaining relationships with loved ones while caregiving.

Regular Check-Ins: This involves scheduling routine calls, video chats, or text exchanges with friends and family to stay connected.

Why It Matters: Staying in touch with loved ones keeps you grounded, reminds you that you're not alone, and combats the feelings of isolation that caregiving can sometimes bring. These connections provide emotional strength and a sense of normalcy amidst your responsibilities.

Action Steps:

- Schedule regular calls, video chats, or text exchanges with friends and family. Set specific days or times so that it becomes a routine you look forward to.

- Share updates about your caregiving journey, but balance these conversations with lighter, uplifting topics that remind you both of the joys of life.

- If time is tight, simplify communication by sending a quick voice note or a cheerful "thinking of you" message.

Example: Set a recurring reminder to call a close friend every Sunday afternoon. Use this time to catch up on life, laugh together, and encourage one another. This small habit can deepen your bond and help you feel supported.

Inspirational Verse: *Proverbs 17:17*—"A friend loves at all times, and a brother is born for a time of adversity." Relationships are a God-given source of strength, especially during challenging seasons.

Plan Social Outings

Why It Matters: Spending time outside your caregiving routine allows you to recharge and gain a fresh perspective. Social outings remind you of the world beyond your caregiving responsibilities and provide opportunities to experience joy and connection.

Action Steps:

- Arrange casual outings like coffee dates, walks, or meals with friends or family members. Keep plans simple and flexible to fit your schedule.

- If an outing isn't possible, consider inviting someone over for tea or a relaxed conversation at home.

- Even short breaks—like a 20-minute walk—can provide a meaningful pause that refreshes your mind and spirit.

Example: Invite a friend to walk around the park one morning. Share stories, laugh, or simply enjoy the beauty of nature together. These moments of connection can provide a refreshing respite during the hectic caregiving season.

Inspirational Verse: *Matthew 11:28*—"Come to me, all you who are weary and burdened, and I will give you rest." Rest isn't just physical—it can also come through moments of connection and joy with others.

Ask for Help

Why It Matters: Loved ones often want to help but may not know how. By asking for and accepting assistance, you create opportunities for others to be a blessing in your life and contribute to your caregiving journey. Sharing the load doesn't diminish your strength—it multiplies it through community.

Action Steps:

- Be specific about the support you need. Instead of saying, "I'm overwhelmed," ask for concrete help, such as running errands, preparing meals, or briefly covering caregiving duties.

- Accept help without guilt, remembering that it builds your relationship and allows others to fulfill their desire to serve.

- Be clear about how their support makes a difference in your life. Express gratitude often, which strengthens bonds.

Example: When a loved one asks how they can help, say, "It would mean so much if you could pick up groceries this week," or "Could you stay with Mom for an hour while I take a walk?" Small contributions from others can provide significant relief.

Inspirational Verse: *Galatians 6:2*—"Carry each other's burdens, and in this way, you will fulfill the law of Christ." By allowing others to help you, you create a beautiful example of mutual care and Christ-like love in action.

By maintaining connections, prioritizing joyful moments, and involving others in your journey, you can nurture the relationships God has given you. These connections not only ease the caregiving burden but also remind you of the love and support that surrounds you, empowering you to continue your journey with grace and strength.

2. Communicate with Your Loved One: This section focuses on understanding your loved one's perspective, setting boundaries, and incorporating quality time in your caregiving relationship.

Understand Their Perspective

Why It Matters: Open communication fosters empathy, helps you better understand your loved one's feelings, and reassures them that they are valued. This mutual understanding strengthens trust and creates a more harmonious caregiving relationship.

Action Steps:

- Ask about their needs, preferences, and concerns regularly. Let them know their voice matters in decisions affecting their care.
- Practice active listening—make eye contact, acknowledge their feelings, and validate their emotions without judgment.
- Reassure them that they are not a burden and that you are committed to providing care with love and respect.

Example: Ask questions like, "What can I do today to make you feel more comfortable?" or "Is there anything you'd like to share about how you're feeling?" These simple yet thoughtful conversations encourage openness and show your commitment to their well-being.

Inspirational Verse: *Philippians 2:4*—"Let each of you look not only to his own interests but also to the interests of others." Understanding their perspective aligns your care with their unique needs and builds a foundation of compassion.

Set Boundaries

Why It Matters: Establishing healthy boundaries prevents caregiver burnout, protects your mental and physical health, and ensures that you can provide sustainable, quality care over time. Boundaries help both you and your loved one understand that self-care is essential, not selfish.

Action Steps:

- Express your needs in kind yet firm language. Be honest about what you can realistically manage while maintaining your well-being.
- Schedule non-negotiable self-care time and communicate this clearly to your loved one.
- Involve others in caregiving when possible, so you can have regular breaks without guilt.

Example: Say, "I need an hour each afternoon to rest and recharge. It's important to me to take care of myself so I can give you my best care afterward." This approach is both considerate and firm, ensuring that your loved one understands the importance of your boundaries.

Inspirational Verse: *Mark 6:31*—"Then, because so many people were coming and going that they did not even have a chance to eat, he said to them, 'Come with me by yourselves to a quiet place and get some rest.'" Even Jesus emphasized the need for rest—your time to recharge is necessary and holy.

Incorporate Quality Time

Why It Matters: Caregiving often focuses on tasks, but intentionally setting aside time to enjoy each other's company nurtures your emotional bond. These moments of connection remind both of you that your relationship goes beyond the caregiving role.

Action Steps:

- Plan activities that your loved one enjoys and that you can do together, such as watching a favorite movie, baking cookies, or working on a puzzle.

- Take time to reminisce by looking through photo albums or sharing stories from the past.

- Focus on creating joyful and meaningful memories, even in small moments.

Example: Dedicate Saturday afternoons to a shared activity like gardening, playing a simple card game, or listening to their favorite music together. These intentional moments of joy and connection can uplift both of you.

Inspirational Verse: *Proverbs 17:17*—"A friend loves at all times, and a brother is born for a time of adversity." By nurturing moments of connection, you reaffirm the love and care that strengthen you both during challenging times.

By prioritizing communication, setting healthy boundaries, and cherishing quality time, you can create a caregiving environment rooted in love and respect. These practices not only improve your loved one's experience but also enhance your own sense of fulfillment and purpose in this sacred role.

3. Build New Supportive Relationships

Join a Caregiver Support Group

Why It Matters:

Caregiving can sometimes feel isolating, but connecting with others who share similar experiences fosters understanding, encouragement, and a sense of community. Support groups provide a safe space where you can express your thoughts without fear of judgment and receive practical advice from those who truly understand your journey.

Action Steps:

1. **Explore Local and Online Groups:**
   - Look for caregiver support groups in your community, such as those hosted by hospitals, senior centers, or faith organizations.
   - Join online forums or virtual groups that offer flexibility and access to a wider network of caregivers.
2. **Participate Actively:**
   - Share your challenges and triumphs openly to build connections with others.
   - Offer support to fellow caregivers by listening and sharing insights from your own experiences.
3. **Commit to Regular Attendance:**
   - Make these meetings a part of your routine to consistently benefit from the shared wisdom and camaraderie.

Examples of Support Groups:

- **Family Caregiver Alliance Support Groups:** Visit car egiver.orgto find resources and support groups tailored to caregivers.
- **The Caregiver Space:** Explore thecaregiverspace.org for a vibrant online community of caregivers sharing their journeys.

Expand Your Social Circle

Why It Matters:

Socializing outside the caregiving world provides a refreshing change, introduces you to new perspectives, and reminds you that life is rich with opportunities for connection and growth. Developing friendships outside of caregiving can help replenish your energy and widen your support network.

Action Steps:

1. **Attend Community Events:**
    - Look for gatherings such as fairs, workshops, or church events to meet like-minded individuals.
    - Consider joining a faith-based small group or ministry to connect with others who share your values.
2. **Pursue Your Interests:**
    - Engage in activities you enjoy, like book clubs, fitness classes, crafting groups, or cooking classes.
    - Use these opportunities to meet new people who share your passions.

3. **Say Yes to Invitations:**

    - Accept invitations from friends or acquaintances, even if you feel hesitant at first. These interactions could lead to meaningful new relationships.

Example:

Join a book club at your local library to discuss literature and connect with others who share your love of reading. Alternatively, sign up for a fitness class, such as yoga or walking groups, to improve your well-being while making new friends.

Inspirational Verse: *Ecclesiastes 4:9-10*—"Two are better than one because they have a good return for their labor: If either of them falls down, one can help the other up."

Building new relationships strengthens your support network and reminds you that you are never truly alone in your caregiving journey.

By participating in caregiver support groups and broadening your social connections, you create opportunities for support, understanding, and personal development. These relationships not only enrich your life but also empower you to navigate the challenges of caregiving with renewed energy and hope.

4. Protect Your Relationships

Avoid Isolation

Why It Matters:

Prolonged isolation can lead to loneliness, emotional fatigue, and even resentment. Staying connected with others helps you maintain a sense of community and prevents you from feeling overwhelmed by caregiving responsibilities. It also reminds you that you are not alone and that there are people who care about your well-being.

Action Steps:

1. **Proactively Reach Out:**

- Take the initiative to connect with friends and family, even when it feels inconvenient or you're tired. Small efforts to maintain these relationships can have a big impact.

2. **Schedule Social Moments:**

   - Plan small interactions throughout your week, such as coffee breaks with a friend, a quick phone call, or a brief walk with a neighbor.

Example:

If your schedule is packed, send a quick text to a loved one saying, "Thinking of you! Let's catch up soon." This simple gesture shows you value the relationship and keeps the connection alive.

Practice Forgiveness

Why It Matters:

Stress can cause misunderstandings or frustrations, but forgiveness is key to restoring harmony and keeping relationships healthy. Letting go of resentment—whether toward yourself or others—frees you from emotional burdens and allows relationships to thrive, even in challenging times.

Action Steps:

1. **Address Conflicts With Empathy:**

   - Approach disagreements calmly and with an open heart. Share your feelings honestly and listen to the other person's perspective without judgment.

2. **Forgive Yourself and Others:**

   - Recognize that everyone, including you, makes mistakes

under stress. Forgiveness creates space for healing and moving forward together.

Example:

If a family member forgot to help with a task, say, "I felt overwhelmed when you couldn't assist me yesterday. Let's find a way to make things easier next time." This approach encourages understanding and co-operation rather than conflict.

Acknowledge Your Emotions

Why It Matters:

Suppressing emotions can lead to strained relationships, increased stress, and even physical health problems. Acknowledging and expressing your feelings allows you to process them in healthy ways, strengthen emotional bonds, and reduce internal tension.

Action Steps:

1. **Share With Trusted Friends or Family Members.**
    - Be open about how you feel, whether it's joy, sadness, frustration, or hope. Letting others in fosters closeness and helps you feel understood.

2. **Journal or Pray for Reflection:**
    - Writing your thoughts in a journal or bringing them to God in prayer provides clarity and peace. It's an opportunity to release burdens and seek guidance.

Example:

Call a friend and say, "I'm feeling overwhelmed today. Do you have a few minutes to talk?" Being vulnerable can lead to meaningful conversations that strengthen your bond.

Inspirational Verse:*Psalm 34:18*—"The Lord is close to the brokenhearted and saves those who are crushed in spirit."
This verse reminds us that even in moments of emotional pain, God is near, offering comfort and strength. Sharing your struggles with loved ones reflects His intention for us to support and uplift one another.

By staying connected, forgiving, and recognizing your emotions, you safeguard your most important relationships. These deliberate actions promote understanding between people, forge enduring relationships, and guarantee that love, empathy, and connection will be there to support you on your caregiving journey.

5. Prioritize Intimate Relationships

Make Time for Your Partner

Why It Matters:

Your relationship with your partner is a cornerstone of emotional stability and mutual support, especially during the demands of caregiving. Prioritizing time together helps you both feel valued and connected, reminding you that your partnership is a source of strength and love.

Action Steps:

1. **Dedicate Uninterrupted Time Daily:**
    - Set aside at least 30 minutes each day to talk, laugh, or simply enjoy each other's company without interruptions.
    - Use this time to share your thoughts, dreams, or even moments of gratitude for one another.
2. **Plan Simple Date Nights:**
    - Arrange intentional moments to nurture your relation-

ship, even if it's just at home. A small effort can reignite intimacy and deepen your bond.

- Avoid distractions such as phones and caregiving tasks during these times.

Example:

Prepare dinner together and enjoy it by candlelight, creating a warm and intimate atmosphere. Use the opportunity to talk about topics unrelated to caregiving, focusing on your shared interests and dreams.

Seek Support Together

Why It Matters:

Facing caregiving challenges as a team not only reduces stress but also strengthens your unity. Working together creates a shared sense of purpose and ensures that neither partner feels isolated in their role.

Action Steps:

1. **Divide Responsibilities:**
    - Communicate openly about how to share caregiving tasks and household duties.
    - Play to each other's strengths when dividing responsibilities, ensuring a balanced approach.
2. **Explore Support Resources Together:**
    - Attend caregiver workshops or join support groups as a couple to gain insights and connect with others who understand your journey.
    - Consider couples counseling or therapy to work through challenges and enhance your partnership.

Example:

Join a local caregiver workshop or attend an online webinar as a couple. Use the experience to learn new strategies, share perspectives, and feel more equipped to tackle challenges together.

Inspirational Verse:*Ephesians 5:33*—"However, each one of you also must love his wife as he loves himself, and the wife must respect her husband."

This verse emphasizes the importance of love and respect in a marriage, reminding you to nurture your relationship even amidst the demands of caregiving.

By prioritizing time with your partner and seeking support as a team, you build a strong, loving, and deeply connected relationship. This intentional focus on your partnership ensures that caregiving challenges are met with unity, and your love remains a source of strength for both of you

6. Celebrate Your Support Network

Express Gratitude

Why It Matters:

Showing gratitude strengthens relationships and encourages those who support you to continue doing so. Acknowledging the contributions of others fosters mutual respect and appreciation, creating a positive and uplifting dynamic within your support network.

Action Steps:

1. **Send Personal Thanks:**
    - Write a heartfelt thank-you note, send a thoughtful text, or give a small gift as a token of appreciation.
    - Be specific about what you're thankful for, so they understand the impact of their help.

2. **Acknowledge Contributions Verbally:**

    - During conversations, take a moment to express gratitude for their efforts, whether big or small.
    - Simple words of thanks can brighten someone's day and reinforce their importance in your life.

Example:

Say, "Your help with grocery shopping last week made a huge difference—thank you so much! I truly appreciate you taking the time to support me."

Show Appreciation

Why It Matters:

Celebrating milestones and moments of joy highlights the positive aspects of your caregiving journey and brings people together. These celebrations remind you and your support network of the good that can be found in even the most challenging circumstances.

Action Steps:

1. **Celebrate Milestones and Achievements:**

    - Host a small gathering to mark a caregiving milestone, such as successfully navigating a tough period or a loved one's recovery progress.
    - Make these occasions meaningful, even if they're simple.

2. **Create Uplifting Memories:**

    - Share moments of joy with your loved ones to build positive associations with your caregiving experience.
    - Use these occasions to strengthen your emotional bonds

and reflect on the support you've received.

Example:

Bake a cake for a sibling who regularly helps out, and spend the evening reminiscing about fond memories. Share laughter and gratitude to deepen your connection and create an uplifting moment.

Inspirational Verse: *1 Thessalonians 5:11*—"Therefore encourage one another and build each other up, just as in fact you are doing." This verse reminds us to celebrate and support one another, recognizing the strength we draw from our shared journey.

By showing gratitude and celebrating your support system, you create a culture of appreciation and unity that bolsters relationships and enriches the caregiving experience. These acts of appreciation not only uplift those around you but also deepen your relationships, ensuring that your caregiving journey is filled with love, connection, and joy.

Final Thought

By nurturing your relationships, you build a vital network of support that helps you thrive as a caregiver. These connections provide emotional sustenance, practical help, and the reassurance that you are not alone in your journey. At its heart, caregiving is a shared experience enriched by the love, understanding, and presence of others.

Take a moment today to reach out, express gratitude, or deepen a connection with someone who matters in your life. Whether it's a heartfelt conversation, a simple act of kindness, or a shared laugh, these moments strengthen the bonds that uplift and sustain you.

John 15:12—"My command is this: Love each other as I have loved you," emphasizing the importance of showing love to others as Christ has shown love to you.

This command emphasizes that love, shown through actions, forms the basis of all significant relationships. By embodying this love in your caregiving journey, you reflect Christ's care and compassion, not just for your loved one but for yourself and your support network as well.

Always remember that you have a strong support system by your side. With faith and love, you can navigate even the most challenging days with grace and strength.

CHAPTER 7

INDULGE IN SMALL JOYS

"You make known to me the path of life; in your presence there is fullness of joy; at your right hand are pleasures forevermore."
Psalm 16:11

Amid the demanding responsibilities of caregiving, it's easy to overlook your own need for joy and personal fulfillment. However, carving out moments to indulge in small joys isn't just a luxury—it's a necessity for your emotional well-being and overall resilience. These seemingly simple moments of happiness can act as a balm for the soul, a reminder of life's beauty, and a source of strength to keep going.

Small joys serve as a refreshing refreshment to a parched soul. They provide balance amidst the challenges of caregiving, helping you maintain a sense of self beyond the tasks and responsibilities that fill your days. These moments allow you to reconnect with your passions, embrace gratitude, and draw closer to the peace that comes from knowing that joy is a gift from God.

Why Small Joys Matter:

- **Emotional Renewal:** A boost in emotional well-being and a reduction in emotional burden can occur even with a brief moment of happiness.
- **Physical Health:** Joy triggers the release of endorphins, which not only reduce stress but also boost the immune system and promote overall well-being, contributing to improved physical health.
- **Perspective:** When you intentionally pause to enjoy life, it helps shift your focus from what's missing to what's meaningful.
- **Connection with God:** experiencing joy is a direct pathway to feeling enveloped in God's blessings and His desire for you to thrive abundantly, even amidst life's trials.

The beauty of small joys lies in their simplicity. A cup of tea on a quiet morning, the warmth of sunlight on your face, a good book, or a favorite song can transform an ordinary moment into something extraordinary. It's not about grand gestures or long vacations but rather about recognizing and embracing the blessings already present in your daily life.

Psalm 16:11 says, "You make known to me the path of life; in your presence there is fullness of joy; at your right hand are pleasures forevermore." This verse reminds us that joy originates from God's presence, and even in the busiest seasons, His gifts of comfort, peace, and delight are within reach.

In this chapter, we will explore ways to incorporate small joys into your routine, discover how these moments can reinvigorate your caregiving journey, and reflect on the deep satisfaction that comes from embracing life's simple pleasures. By prioritizing these moments, you'll not only find renewed strength for caregiving but also experience the fullness of life that God has prepared for you.

1. Rediscover Activities You Enjoy

Hobbies and Passions

Why It Matters:
Engaging in hobbies you love is a way to reconnect with your identity beyond caregiving. It provides a much-needed creative outlet, reduces stress, and reminds you of the joy and fulfillment that come from doing something just for yourself. These activities are not selfish—they're vital to maintaining your well-being and allowing you to continue caregiving with energy and a positive mindset.

Examples:

- **Art and Craft:**
  Explore creative pursuits like painting, knitting, scrapbooking, or making handmade cards. Engaging in artistic activities is therapeutic and provides a sense of accomplishment.
  Example: Maria, a caregiver, rediscovered her love for painting watercolors in the evenings after her caregiving duties. She called it her "peaceful pause," a time to quiet her mind and find calm amidst her busy day.

- **Gardening:**
  Whether it's tending to flowers, growing vegetables, or simply watering potted plants, gardening offers a calming escape. The act of nurturing plants reflects the care you give to others, reminding you of life's growth and beauty.
  Example: Spending 15 minutes each morning watering her plants became a sacred routine for Lila, who found peace in the simplicity of watching her garden flourish.

- **Reading:**
  Escape into a novel, dive into a devotional, or explore a self-help book that uplifts your spirit. Reading is both an educational and emotional retreat.
  Example: Consider joining a book club to connect with others who share your love for reading. Engaging in discussions about books provides both intellectual stimulation and social interaction.

Inspirational Verse:

Proverbs 17:22—"A cheerful heart is good medicine, but a crushed spirit dries up the bones." Finding joy in your hobbies nourishes your spirit, bringing vitality and strength to your caregiving journey.

Music and Movies

Why It Matters:

Music and movies have a unique power to elevate your mood, reduce stress, and transport you to a more positive emotional space. They provide an instant escape from the pressures of caregiving, allowing you to relax and recharge.

Examples:

- **Music:**
    - Listen to uplifting songs, classical pieces, or nostalgic tunes that evoke happy memories.
    - Create a playlist of your favorite songs to play during caregiving tasks, turning routine moments into enjoyable experiences.
      Example: Sarah found that playing her favorite worship music while preparing meals brought a sense of peace and gratitude to her day.
- **Movies:**
    - Watch a feel-good movie or a lighthearted comedy to boost your mood. Laughter releases endorphins, which help reduce stress and elevate your spirit.
      Example: After a particularly challenging day, David watched an old favorite comedy, laughing until his sides hurt, and felt rejuvenated to face the next day.

Inspirational Verse:

Psalm 95:1—"Come, let us sing for joy to the Lord; let us shout aloud to the Rock of our salvation." Let music and moments of joy remind you of God's presence and the beauty of life.

Exercise and Movement

Why It Matters:

Physical activity is not only beneficial for your body but also crucial for enhancing mental clarity, emotional well-being, and spiritual balance. Movement releases endorphins, enhances mental clarity, and lifts your mood. It's a way to care for the body God has given you while finding moments of peace and joy in the process.

Examples:

- **Yoga:**
  Take a yoga class or follow a video at home to combine stretching, mindfulness, and relaxation. This practice helps you center yourself and release physical tension.
  Example: Emily discovered a 15-minute yoga routine online that became her daily morning ritual, setting a calm and positive tone for the day.

- **Dancing:**
  Turn on your favorite upbeat song and dance around your living room. It's a quick way to boost your mood and energize your body.
  Example: Before bedtime, Jenny danced with her toddler to their favorite music, creating moments of pure joy while staying active.

- **Walking:**
  Take a walk in a nearby park or around your neighborhood. Use this time to appreciate the beauty of nature, reflect, and pray.
  Example: John set aside 20 minutes every evening to walk in the park, finding peace in the sound of rustling leaves and birdsong.

Inspirational Verse:

1 Corinthians 6:19-20—"Your body is a temple of the Holy Spirit. .. glorify God in your body." Caring for your body through movement is an act of worship, honoring the gift of life God has given you.

Rediscovering activities you love helps you maintain balance and joy, even in the busiest seasons of caregiving. By prioritizing hobbies, music, movies, and physical movement, you not only nurture your emotional well-being but also invite God's presence into your moments of rest and renewal. These small joys are gifts that sustain and empower you for the journey ahead.

2. Create a "Joy List."

Write It Down

Why It Matters:
A joy list is a simple yet powerful tool to remind you of the little things that brighten your day, especially during moments when life feels overwhelming. Writing these joys down helps you focus on the positive and gives you practical ideas for self-care when you need a quick pick-me-up. It's a tangible way to keep gratitude and happiness within reach, even amidst challenges.

Action Steps:

1. **List the Things That Make You Happy:**
    - Reflect on small activities, treats, or moments that bring you joy.
    - Include sensory delights, like the aroma of a favorite candle, the taste of a treat, or the feel of warm sunlight.
2. **Make Your Joy List Visible:**
    - Write your list on colorful paper or in a special notebook

and place it somewhere you'll see daily—on your fridge, desk, or bedside table.

- Alternatively, create a digital version on your phone or tablet for easy access.

Example Joys to Add:

- Enjoying a cup of tea or coffee in a cozy spot.
- Watching a sunrise or sunset.
- Lighting a scented candle with your favorite fragrance.
- Listening to birds sing or the sound of rain.
- Taking five minutes to stretch or meditate.

Incorporate Joys Daily

Why It Matters:
Small moments of joy, when woven into your daily routine, can uplift your mood, reduce stress, and provide a sense of calm amidst a busy caregiving schedule. By intentionally including these joys, you cultivate a habit of self-care and gratitude.

Examples:

1. **Start Your Day with a Moment of Joy:**
    - Savor your favorite coffee or tea while sitting in a peaceful corner, reflecting on your blessings.
    - Open your window to feel the morning breeze and listen to the world waking up.

2. **Pause to Appreciate Beauty:**
   - Take a moment to admire the colors of the sky during sunset.
   - Keep a small vase of fresh flowers or a potted plant nearby to enjoy the beauty of nature.
3. **Relax with Intentional Comforts:**
   - Diffuse a soothing essential oil, like lavender or citrus, while reading or journaling.
   - Wrap yourself in a soft blanket and watch a favorite movie or read a good book.

Inspirational Verse:

Psalm 118:24—"This is the day that the Lord has made; let us rejoice and be glad in it."

Each day is a gift, filled with opportunities to experience joy. Your joy list is a way to honor God's blessings by savoring the little things that make life beautiful.

By creating and using a joy list, you give yourself permission to prioritize happiness and gratitude in your daily life. These small acts of joy not only recharge your spirit but also serve as a reminder that even in the busiest or most challenging moments, God's goodness is all around you.

3. Practice Gratitude

Daily Gratitude Journal

Why It Matters:

Gratitude has the power to transform your perspective by shifting your focus from challenges to blessings. Even in difficult times, reflecting on what you're thankful for can bring a sense of peace, joy, and hope. A gratitude journal serves as a tangible reminder of the good in your life, helping you navigate caregiving with a more positive outlook.

Action Steps:

1. **Set Aside Five Minutes Daily:**
    - Each day, write down three things you're grateful for. These could be small, like the warmth of sunlight, a good cup of coffee, or a moment of laughter with a loved one.
2. **Reflect on Small Moments:**
    - Pay attention to little joys, like a kind smile, a meaningful conversation, or a moment of stillness. Writing them down helps you savor these blessings.

Example:

In your journal, you might write:

- "I'm thankful for the sound of birds singing this morning."
- "Grateful for my friend's encouraging text today."
- "Appreciative of the quiet time I had to read this evening."

Inspirational Verse:

Psalm 107:1—"Give thanks to the Lord, for He is good; His love endures forever." Reflecting on God's enduring love can inspire deep gratitude, even in challenging moments.

Gratitude in Action

Why It Matters:

Expressing gratitude not only enhances your own sense of positivity but also strengthens your relationships and spreads joy to others. When you show appreciation for the kindness of others, you deepen your connection and inspire a culture of thankfulness.

Action Steps:

1. **Send Thank-You Notes:**
    - Take time to write a note, send a text, or even call someone to thank them for their support or kindness.
2. **Acknowledge Kindness Verbally:**
    - In daily interactions, express your appreciation for acts of kindness, no matter how small.
    - Practice saying thank you sincerely and often—it's a simple act that has a big impact.

Example:

If a family member helps you with caregiving tasks, say, "I really appreciate your help with dinner last night. It made my day so much easier."

Inspirational Verse:

1 Thessalonians 5:18—"Give thanks in all circumstances; for this is the will of God in Christ Jesus for you." This verse reminds us to cultivate a heart of gratitude, regardless of the challenges we face, as a reflection of God's goodness.

By practicing gratitude, both in reflection and action, you create a cycle of positivity that uplifts your spirit and strengthens your relationships. It's a simple yet powerful way to honor God's blessings and bring light into your caregiving journey.

4. Treat Yourself

Pamper Days

Why It Matters:
Caring for yourself is not indulgence—it's essential. Pamper days serve as a reminder that your well-being is just as important as the care you provide for others. They help you recharge physically and emotionally, enabling you to return to your caregiving duties with renewed energy and focus.

Examples:

1. **Enjoy a Relaxing Bath:**

    - Run a long bubble bath with soothing scents like lavender or eucalyptus. Add calming music or soft candlelight to enhance the experience.

2. **Try a DIY Spa Experience:**

    - Apply a facial mask, give yourself a manicure, or try aromatherapy at home. These simple self-care acts can help you feel refreshed and nurtured.

3. **Indulge in a Spa Day:**

    - If time allows, visit a local spa for a massage, facial, or pedicure. Letting someone else care for you is a powerful act of self-love.

Example:

Sarah, a caregiver, turned her bathroom into a spa for an evening. She lit candles, played instrumental music, and soaked in a bubble bath, emerging calm and rejuvenated.

Inspirational Verse:

Matthew 11:28—"Come to me, all you who are weary and burdened, and I will give you rest." Allow yourself moments of rest and relaxation, trusting that self-care honors God's desire for your peace and renewal.

Small Rewards

Why It Matters:

Celebrating small wins or simply treating yourself to something special boosts morale and keeps you motivated. These small rewards act as reminders that your efforts matter, and they give you something to look forward to during your caregiving journey.

Examples:

1. **Lift Your Mood With Fresh Flowers:**

    - Buy a bouquet of flowers for your home. The vibrant colors and fragrance can brighten your space and uplift your spirit.

2. **Reward Yourself With Something Special:**

    - Order a new book you've been wanting to read, a cozy blanket to relax with, or a special snack you've been craving. These small pleasures can make a big difference in your day.

3. **Celebrate Small Wins:**

    - Acknowledge accomplishments, like completing a particularly hard day or overcoming a challenge, with a treat or a moment of reflection and gratitude.

Example:
After a challenging week, Lisa treated herself to her favorite latte and a new journal, savoring the moment and reflecting on her progress.

Inspirational Verse:
Ecclesiastes 3:13—"That each of them may eat and drink, and find satisfaction in all their toil—this is the gift of God." Celebrating the fruits of your labor, no matter how small, is a way of embracing the joy God intends for you.

By treating yourself, whether through pampering or small rewards, you nurture your own joy and well-being. These moments of self-care remind you that your happiness is just as important as the love and care you provide to others. When you prioritize yourself, you honor the balance that sustains your caregiving journey.

5. Connect with Nature

Why It Matters:

Immersing yourself in nature's embrace has a profound calming and grounding effect, serving as a mental reset button that rejuvenates your spirit and restores clarity to your mind. It offers a chance to step away from daily caregiving demands, allowing you to experience peace, clarity, and connection with God's creation. Nature reminds us of God's majesty and the beauty of life, even in the simplest details.

Examples:

1. **Take a Stroll in the Park:**
    - Walk among trees, along a lake, or down a quiet path. Let the sights, sounds, and scents of nature refresh your senses.
2. **Step Into Your Backyard for Fresh Air:**
    - Even a few minutes outside can make a difference. Stand barefoot on the grass, breathe deeply, and feel the sun or breeze on your skin.
3. **Notice the Beauty Around You:**
    - Pause to appreciate the little details: blooming flowers, rustling leaves, birdsong, or the colors of the sky during sunrise or sunset.
4. **Spend Quiet Time in a Scenic Spot:**
    - Sit by a lake, under a tree, or on a park bench. Use this time for reflection, prayer, or simply enjoying the stillness.

Testimonial:

After feeling overwhelmed with her caregiving responsibilities, Michelle started taking a short walk each evening in her neighborhood. She found that listening to the rustling leaves and watching the sunset became her sanctuary—a time to reset and attain peace before returning home.

Inspirational Verse:

Psalm 19:1—"The heavens declare the glory of God; the skies proclaim the work of his hands."
This verse reminds us that all of creation reflects God's glory, inviting us to pause and marvel at His handiwork.

By connecting with nature, you allow its tranquility to calm your heart and mind. These moments in God's creation can restore your perspective, renew your energy, and provide a gentle reminder of His presence and love in your caregiving journey.

6. Schedule Mini Getaways

Day Trips

Why It Matters:
Short breaks, even if just for a few hours, offer a much-needed mental reset and a refreshing change of scenery. They allow you to step outside your routine, experience a sense of adventure, and recharge your spirit without requiring significant time or effort.

Examples:

1. **Visit a Local Botanical Garden:**

- Stroll through beautifully maintained gardens, breathe in the fragrant flowers, and immerse yourself in the calming atmosphere of nature.

2. **Explore a Museum:**
   - Take a trip to a nearby art gallery, history museum, or cultural center to experience something inspiring and thought-provoking.
3. **Discover New Spots in Your Area:**
   - Try a new café, wander through a quaint bookstore, or visit a nearby nature trail you've never explored.

Example:
Emily planned a spontaneous day trip to a lakeside park just 30 minutes away. She brought a picnic, enjoyed the serene views, and returned home feeling refreshed and uplifted.

Virtual Getaways

Why It Matters:
When it's difficult to leave home, virtual tours and travel experiences can provide a creative way to escape your routine. These digital adventures allow you to explore the world, experience beauty, and feel inspired, all from the comfort of your home.

Examples:

1. **Take Online Museum Tours:**
   - Visit world-famous destinations like the Louvre, the British Museum, or the Smithsonian through their vir-

tual platforms.

2. **Experience Scenic Beauty Virtually:**
    - Explore breathtaking destinations like the Swiss Alps, the Great Barrier Reef, or Japan's cherry blossoms through virtual tours or YouTube videos.
3. **Watch Travel Documentaries:**
    - Immerse yourself in a new culture or landscape by watching documentaries that showcase the wonders of the world.

Example:
Sarah couldn't leave home due to her caregiving duties, but she set aside an evening to take a virtual tour of Italy's Amalfi Coast. She paired it with Italian snacks and music, making the experience both fun and rejuvenating.

Inspirational Verse:

Matthew 6:26—"Look at the birds of the air; they do not sow or reap or store away in barns, and yet your heavenly Father feeds them. Are you not much more valuable than they?"
This verse reminds us of God's care for His creation and His desire for us to find peace and rest, even in life's busiest seasons.

By scheduling mini getaways—whether physical or virtual—you give yourself permission to step away, recharge, and rediscover the joy of new experiences. These brief escapes, whether physical day trips or virtual experiences, can restore your energy by offering a mental reset and a fresh perspective, helping you approach your caregiving responsibilities with renewed strength, clarity, and a sense of rejuvenation.

7. Engage in Mindful Moments

Mindfulness Practices

Why It Matters:
It's easy to become engrossed in worries about the past or future amidst the hustle of caregiving. Mindfulness invites you to anchor yourself in the present moment, reducing stress and helping you appreciate the beauty of now. Practicing mindfulness fosters calmness, clarity, and gratitude, enhancing your emotional resilience.

Examples:

1. **Focus on Your Breath:**
    - Spend five minutes each day focusing on your breathing. Inhale deeply, hold for a moment, and exhale slowly. This simple exercise can calm your mind and center your thoughts.
2. **Observe Your Surroundings:**
    - Take a few moments to notice the details around you—the colors, textures, sounds, and smells. Observing your environment with curiosity helps ground you in the present.
3. **Meditate Using a Guided App or Prayer-Based Meditation:**

- Use an app like Calm or Headspace for a brief guided meditation session. For a spiritual approach, engage in prayer-based meditation, focusing on God's presence and promises.

Example:

Before starting her day, Lisa spends five minutes sitting by her window, focusing on her breath and observing the rustling leaves and morning sunlight. This practice helps her feel calm and ready to face the day.

Inspirational Verse:

Isaiah 26:3—"You will keep in perfect peace those whose minds are steadfast, because they trust in you." Mindfulness, rooted in trust and focus on God, invites His perfect peace into your heart.

Savor the Moment

Why It Matters:

Immersing yourself fully in small pleasures can transform ordinary moments into extraordinary ones. Savoring these experiences enriches your joy, reminds you of life's blessings, and helps you feel more connected to the present.

Examples:

1. **Savor Your Morning Coffee or Tea:**
    - Take time to truly enjoy the aroma, warmth, and flavor of your drink. Sit quietly and let this simple act of indulgence set a positive tone for your day.
2. **Spend Uninterrupted Time With a Pet or Loved One:**
    - Cuddle your pet, stroke their fur, and feel their love and

comfort. Or, spend a few quiet moments with a loved one, enjoying their presence without distractions.

3. **Relish a Favorite Snack or Activity:**
   - Slowly enjoy a favorite snack or dessert, paying attention to the taste and texture. Or, engage in an activity you love, giving it your full attention.

Example:
After her caregiving tasks, Maria takes 10 minutes to savor a piece of dark chocolate with a cup of tea. She focuses on the flavors and allows herself to feel gratitude for this small treat.

Inspirational Verse:
Psalm 46:10—"Be still, and know that I am God." Savoring the moment is an act of stillness that allows you to experience God's presence and peace in everyday life.

By engaging in mindful moments, you invite peace and joy into your day. These practices help you stay present, appreciate the small blessings, and nurture your emotional well-being, equipping you to approach caregiving with a calm and steady heart.

8. Foster Positive Connections

Social Interactions

Why It Matters:
Human connection is a powerful antidote to stress and loneliness. Spending time with others—whether through laughter, shared meals, or meaningful conversations—reminds you of the joy in companion-

ship and the strength found in community. Positive social interactions rejuvenate your spirit, providing emotional support and moments of genuine happiness.

Examples:

1. **Share a Meal With a Friend:**
   - Invite a friend over or meet at a favorite restaurant to enjoy a meal together. Good food and good company create a relaxing, joyful atmosphere.
2. **Call Someone Who Makes You Laugh:**
   - Reach out to a loved one whose sense of humor consistently brightens your day. A few minutes of laughter can ease stress and lift your mood.
3. **Join a Club or Group:**
   - Find a group that aligns with your interests, like a book club, fitness class, or volunteer organization. Connecting with like-minded individuals helps you build new relationships and rekindle passions.

Example:

Jessica joined a local gardening club, where she found a community of people who shared her love of plants. Weekly meetups became her sanctuary, offering her companionship and a creative outlet.

Inspirational Verse:

Hebrews 10:24-25—"And let us consider how we may spur one another on toward love and good deeds, not giving up meeting together, as some are in the habit of doing, but encouraging one another." Social connections are opportunities to uplift and inspire one another, as God intended.

Share Joy With Your Loved One

Why It Matters:
Positive shared activities strengthen your bond with your loved one, fostering closeness and creating joyful memories to cherish. These moments go beyond caregiving tasks, reminding both of you of the love and connection at the heart of your relationship.

Examples:

1. **Watch a Comedy Together:**
   - Pick a lighthearted movie or show that makes you both laugh. Laughter not only reduces stress but also creates a shared moment of joy.
2. **Bake Cookies or Cook a Meal Together:**
   - Involve your loved one in simple activities like baking or preparing a favorite dish. The process of working together can be fun and fulfilling.
3. **Listen to Their Favorite Music:**
   - Play songs that bring back good memories for them. Share the experience by dancing, singing along, or simply listening together.
4. **Reminisce About Happy Memories:**
   - Look through photo albums or talk about cherished moments from the past. Reflecting on good times can

bring smiles and strengthen your emotional connection.

Example:

Michael and his elderly father spent an afternoon listening to old jazz records. They shared stories about the music, laughed, and created a memory that Michael treasured long after.

Inspirational Verse:

Romans 12:10—"Be devoted to one another in love. Honor one another above yourselves." Sharing joy with your loved one reflects the love and honor God calls us to demonstrate in our relationships.

By fostering positive connections—whether with friends, family, or your loved one—you create a supportive network filled with love, joy, and emotional well-being, enhancing your resilience and enriching your caregiving journey. These relationships remind you of life's beauty and offer strength to navigate the challenges of caregiving with hope and gratitude.

9. Celebrate Achievements

Why It Matters:

Celebrating your achievements, both big and small, is essential for maintaining motivation and recognizing the value of your hard work. As a caregiver, it's easy to overlook your accomplishments because you're so focused on others. Taking time to acknowledge your efforts reinforces your sense of purpose, boosts your morale, and reminds you that your dedication makes a meaningful difference.

Examples:

1. **Treat Yourself After Completing a Challenging Task:**
    - Reward yourself with something special after accomplishing a difficult caregiving responsibility. This could be a favorite snack, a relaxing bath, or a small gift you've been wanting.
2. **Share Your Accomplishments With Loved Ones:**
    - Let family or friends know about your achievements, no matter how small they may seem. Sharing your success invites others to celebrate with you and offers an opportunity for encouragement.
3. **Create a "Win Jar" or Journal:**
    - Write down your accomplishments, no matter how minor, and place them in a jar or log them in a journal. Reflect on these wins regularly to see how far you've come.

Inspirational Verse:

Philippians 4:13—"I can do all things through Him who strengthens me." This verse reminds you that your achievements, no matter how challenging, are possible with God's guidance and strength.

By celebrating your achievements, you not only honor your hard work and perseverance but also acknowledge the value of your dedication and the impact of your accomplishments in the caregiving journey. These moments of recognition not only uplift your spirit but also serve as reminders of your capability and dedication in the caregiving journey. Treat yourself, share your success, and know that each step forward is worth celebrating.

10. Keep Things Simple

Why It Matters:

Life's simplest joys are often the most meaningful and easiest to incorporate into your daily routine. They don't require elaborate plans or significant time commitments, making them accessible even during busy caregiving days. Embracing simplicity helps you find peace and gratitude in the little moments, reminding you that joy is always within reach.

Examples:

1. **Take Five Minutes to Stretch and Breathe Deeply**
    - Start your morning or take a quick pause during the day to stretch your body and take deep, intentional breaths. This simple practice helps release tension and restores your focus.
2. **Listen to an Uplifting Podcast While You Cook or Clean:**
    - Turn routine tasks into opportunities for inspiration by listening to an encouraging podcast or an audiobook.
3. **Watch the Rain With a Warm Blanket and a Cup of**

Tea:

- When it's raining, take a moment to sit by a window, cozy up with a blanket, and enjoy the soothing sound of the rain with your favorite warm drink.

4. **Light a Scented Candle While You Journal or Read:**
    - The calming glow and fragrance can create a peaceful atmosphere that elevates an ordinary moment into something special.
5. **Step Outside for Fresh Air:**
    - Spend a few minutes outside, even if it's just standing in your backyard or taking a short walk around the block. Feel the breeze, observe the sky, and let the simplicity of nature refresh you.

Inspirational Verse:

Matthew 6:34—"Therefore do not worry about tomorrow, for tomorrow will worry about itself. Each day has enough trouble of its own." Keeping things simple allows you to focus on the present and find peace in the here and now, trusting God with the rest.

By keeping things simple, you effortlessly integrate joy into your daily life, making it a natural and accessible part of your routine. These small, intentional moments of simplicity help you stay grounded, refreshed, and ready to navigate the caregiving journey with grace and gratitude.

Final Thought

Indulging in small joys serves as a powerful reminder of the beauty and blessings that exist in everyday life, even during the most challenging times. These moments of happiness do more than simply lift your mood—they rejuvenate your spirit, offering a sense of balance and peace that helps you navigate the caregiving journey with renewed energy and positivity.

Start by identifying one small thing you can do for yourself today, whether it's savoring a quiet cup of tea, taking a short walk, or pausing to appreciate a moment of stillness. Commit to making it a part of your routine, knowing that these simple acts of self-care are essential for your well-being. You deserve to feel joy, not just for yourself but also as a way to replenish and sustain your capacity to care for others with love and compassion, creating a cycle of well-being and kindness.

John 15:11—"I have told you this so that my joy may be in you and that your joy may be complete."

Let this verse remind you that God desires for you to experience His joyfulness, even amidst the challenges of caregiving. By embracing small joys, you honor His gift of life and find the strength to continue your journey with grace and gratitude.

CHAPTER 8

DAY-OF-EXAM TIPS

"Have I not commanded you? Be strong and courageous. Do not be afraid; do not be discouraged, for the Lord your God will be with you wherever you go."
Joshua 1:9

The day you've been working toward is finally here. After months of studying, practicing, and dedicating yourself to mastering the material, it's time to take the AGPCNP exam and showcase your hard-earned knowledge and skills.

Success on exam day is not just about knowing the material—it is about effectively managing your time, energy, and mindset to optimize performance. A clear plan can help you navigate the day with focus and confidence, ensuring that your preparation translates into the best results possible. This chapter offers practical strategies to help you stay calm, composed, and focused, maximizing your performance and maintaining a positive outlook throughout the exam process.

Success on exam day is not only about mastering the material but also about efficiently managing your time, energy, and mindset to optimize performance.

- **Physical Readiness:** To stay alert and energized, ensure you get a good night's sleep, eat a nutritious breakfast, and do some light stretching. Well-rested and nourished bodies help optimize focus and stamina.

- **Mental Clarity:** A calm and organized mind is better equipped to handle the pressure of the exam environment.

- **Emotional Balance:** Managing nerves and maintaining confidence can prevent stress from undermining your efforts.

- **Spiritual Strength:** Drawing on your faith can provide peace, encouragement, and the assurance that you're not alone.

The morning of your exam sets the tone for the entire day. A well-thought-out routine can minimize stress and maximize focus:

- Wake up early to give yourself plenty of time to prepare for the exam.

- Eat a balanced breakfast with brain-boosting foods like whole grains, fruit, and protein.

- Double-check your materials, including your ID, exam confirmation, and any allowed items.

- Dress comfortably, keeping in mind the environment of the

exam center when selecting your attire.

Emotional Readiness:

It's common to experience nervousness, but it's essential not to let anxiety overwhelm you. To stay centered and focused, use practical strategies such as deep breathing, positive self-talk, and visualization. Remind yourself of the hard work you've put into preparing and trust in your ability to succeed.

Spiritual Encouragement:

Before the exam, take a moment to pray, meditate, or reflect to center yourself and draw strength from your faith. Remember that you are supported and guided by a higher power.

Before heading to the exam center, pause to pray, meditate, or reflect. Draw on God's promises for strength and guidance, such as the comforting words of Isaiah 41:10:

"Fear not, for I am with you; be not dismayed, for I am your God; I will strengthen you, I will help you, I will uphold you with my righteous right hand."

These words serve as a powerful reminder that you are never alone in facing challenges—God is by your side, providing strength and support every step of the way.

In this chapter, you'll find detailed tips for managing your time during the exam, strategies for tackling challenging questions, and ways to maintain your confidence throughout the day. With a clear plan, a calm heart, and trust in God, you'll be ready to give your best and embrace this moment as a testament to your hard work and dedication.

1. Prepare a Detailed Checklist

Approaching exam day with a well-organized plan can significantly reduce stress and set the stage for success. By preparing a detailed checklist, you ensure that you're fully equipped and ready to handle any surprises. This small yet powerful step helps you feel more confident and in control, allowing you to focus entirely on the task at hand—your exam.

Including backup items on your checklist is crucial for exam readiness. These items serve as your safety net, preparing you for unexpected situations that might otherwise disrupt your focus and performance. Whether it's a pen running out of ink, a forgotten tool, or an issue with time management, having backups ensures you remain calm and adaptable, no matter what challenges arise.

Why Backup Items Are Essential:

Backup items allow you to stay in control during unforeseen situations. A small oversight, like a malfunctioning watch or a misplaced pen, can quickly escalate into stress if you don't have a solution ready. By including these items, you eliminate unnecessary worry and keep your attention where it belongs—on doing your best.

Example:

Jane's watch battery unexpectedly died during her exam, but because she brought a backup analog watch, she could continue tracking her time without stress. This proactive preparation helped her complete the exam on schedule and with confidence.

Taking the time to anticipate and prepare for potential issues with a detailed checklist, including backup items, reflects both diligence and readiness. This approach not only minimizes stress but also ensures you can focus fully on your performance, knowing you've planned for success.

Essentials to Bring

- **Government-Issued ID:**
    - Double-check that the name on your ID matches your

exam registration. Any discrepancies could cause delays or complications.

- **Example:** Sarah realized the night before her exam that her driver's license had expired. By preparing a checklist early, she avoided panic and brought her passport instead.

- **Admission Ticket:**
  - As per exam requirements, print your ticket ahead of time or have it ready digitally. Keep it in a folder or a dedicated pocket in your bag for easy access.
- **Snacks and Water:**
  - Pack light, non-messy snacks such as granola bars, fruit, or nuts to keep your energy up during breaks.
  - To stay hydrated, you must bring a reusable water bottle. Check if the exam center has restrictions on bringing water bottles into the room.
  - **Example:** Mark packed a small apple and almonds for his break, giving him the energy boost he needed to stay sharp during the second half of his exam.
- **Comfortable Clothing:**
  - Dress in layers to adapt to varying room temperatures. Wear comfortable, non-restrictive clothing to avoid distractions.
  - **Example:** Emma wore a light sweater over her T-shirt,

which she easily removed when the exam room warmed up.

- **Medication or Supplies:**
    - If you need specific items, such as prescription glasses, an inhaler, or medication, make sure they are in your bag and easily accessible.

Backup Items

While the document highlights the importance of including backup items, it's equally important to understand why they are essential for exam readiness. Backup items safeguard against unexpected challenges, such as a malfunctioning tool or a last-minute oversight, that could otherwise disrupt your focus and performance.

Why They're Essential:

- **Preparedness:** Unexpected situations, like a pen running out of ink or a watch malfunctioning, can create unnecessary stress during an exam. Having backups ensures you're ready to handle such scenarios calmly.
- **Focus Maintenance:** Knowing you have extra supplies allows you to stay focused on the exam itself, rather than worrying about potential mishaps.
- **Adaptability:** Backup items demonstrate proactive planning and allow you to adapt seamlessly to any surprises.

Example:

Imagine a pen suddenly stops working in the middle of the exam. Without a backup, you may feel flustered and lose valuable time.

However, with an extra pen at hand, you can quickly resume your work without distraction, keeping your momentum intact.

Including backup items on your checklist ensures you're fully prepared for anything, reinforcing your confidence and allowing you to approach the exam with a calm and composed mindset.

- **Extra Pen or Pencil:**
    - If the exam allows you to bring writing tools, pack extras. A pen running out of ink or a broken pencil shouldn't derail your focus.
- **Watch or Timer:**
    - Use an analog or silent digital watch if allowed. Tracking time discreetly helps you pace yourself without relying solely on the exam center's clock.

Proverbs 21:5:

This verse highlights that careful planning and diligence pave the way for success and abundance, contrasting with hastiness that can lead to shortcomings. It underscores the importance of thorough preparation for achieving favorable outcomes.

This verse beautifully underscores the importance of preparation and careful planning. Taking the time to organize yourself before exam day ensures a smoother experience, reducing anxiety and creating an environment where you can thrive.

Inspiration for Success:

Preparing a checklist isn't just about avoiding mishaps—it's about stepping into the exam room with confidence, knowing you've done everything possible to be ready. Picture this moment as part of the diligence and discipline you've cultivated throughout your journey.

You've planned, you've prepared, and now it's time to perform with assurance.

So, tonight, take a few minutes to review your checklist, pack your bag, and pray for calm and focus. You've got this—and with preparation and faith, you're ready to shine.

2. Eat a Nourishing Breakfast

Fueling your body is just as important as preparing your mind for exam day. The food you eat on the morning of your exam plays a critical role in stabilizing your energy levels, keeping your mind sharp, and ensuring you stay focused throughout the test. A balanced breakfast can prevent distractions caused by hunger and help you maintain steady performance during this important moment.

Why It Matters:

- **Energy Stability:** A nourishing breakfast provides the fuel your body needs to sustain energy levels, avoiding the dips and crashes that can come with poor food choices.
- **Mental Focus:** Nutrient-dense foods enhance brain function, helping you think clearly and recall information more effectively.
- **Hunger Prevention:** Eating a satisfying meal prevents hunger from becoming a distraction during the exam, allowing you to focus fully on your tasks.

Examples:

1. **Protein-Packed Option:**
    - Scrambled eggs, whole-grain toast, and avocado slices make a well-rounded breakfast packed with protein, healthy fats, and complex carbs for sustained energy.

2. **Quick Option:**

  - Blend a smoothie with fruits, spinach, protein powder, and almond milk. For extra nutrients, add a tablespoon of nut butter or chia seeds.

3. **Snacks to Avoid:**

  - Avoid sugary pastries, donuts, and heavy, greasy foods, which can cause a mid-morning energy crash or leave you feeling sluggish.

Inspirational Tip:

Think of your breakfast as the foundation for a successful day. Just as a car needs fuel to run smoothly, your body and brain need the right nutrients to perform at their best. By starting your day with a nourishing meal, you're giving yourself the physical and mental edge to approach your exam with clarity and focus.

Inspirational Verse:

1 Corinthians 10:31—"So whether you eat or drink or whatever you do, do it all for the glory of God."

Eating well honors the body God has given you and ensures you are prepared to give your best effort on this important day.

3. Arrive Early

Giving yourself extra time to arrive and settle into the testing environment can set the tone for a calm and focused exam day. By arriving early, you avoid the stress of rushing and give yourself the opportunity to acclimate, organize, and mentally prepare for the task ahead.

Action Steps:

1. **Plan Your Route:**

  - Map out the testing location in advance. Check for traffic updates, parking availability, or public transit schedules to ensure you know the fastest and most reliable route.

- Consider doing a trial run to the location a day or two before the exam to familiarize yourself with the route and the surroundings.

2. **Arrive 30 Minutes Early:**

    - Use this time to check in, find your seat, and organize your belongings.

    - Spend a few moments calming your nerves with deep breaths, prayer, or positive affirmations before the exam begins.

    - **Example:** Sarah arrived at her testing center early, giving her time to review her key notes and pray for peace before entering the exam room.

Why It Matters:

- **Reduces Stress:** Arriving early eliminates the rush and panic of being late, giving you a calm and composed start to the exam. It eliminates the anxiety of rushing, ensuring you start the exam feeling calm, prepared, and focused.

- **Prepares Your Mind:** Extra time allows you to mentally shift gears and focus fully on the task ahead.

- **Adapts to the Environment:** Getting familiar with the testing space can boost your comfort and confidence during the exam.

Inspirational Verse:

Psalm 119:105—"Your word is a lamp to my feet and a light to my path."

This verse reminds us of the importance of preparation and God's guidance in every step of our journey. Just as His Word illuminates the path before us, careful planning and arriving early ensure a smooth and confident start to your exam day.

Encouragement:

By arriving early, you set yourself up for success with a clear mind and steady heart. Take this time to pause, reflect, and remind yourself that you are ready for this moment. You've done the work, and with faith and preparation, you're equipped to excel.

4. Relaxation Techniques

Calming your mind and body before the exam is essential for maintaining focus and performing at your best. Stress and anxiety can hinder your ability to think clearly, but incorporating simple relaxation techniques can help you stay centered, confident, and ready to succeed.

Deep Breathing Exercises

Why It Helps:

Controlled breathing lowers stress by activating the body's relaxation response. It increases oxygen flow to the brain, improving focus and mental clarity and helping the person feel grounded and in control.

How to Practice:

1. **Inhale Deeply:**

    - Breathe in deeply through your nose for four counts, filling your lungs fully.

2. **Hold Your Breath**

- Hold your breath for four counts, allowing the oxygen to circulate through your body.

3. **Exhale Slowly:**

   - Release your breath slowly through your mouth for six counts, imagining stress leaving your body.

4. **Repeat:**

   - Perform this cycle three to five times or until you feel calmer.

Example: Before entering the exam room, pause for a moment and practice deep breathing. This simple exercise helps you let go of nervous tension and approach the test with a steady mind.

Visualization of Success

Why It Helps:

Visualization is a powerful technique that reinforces a positive mindset. By imagining yourself confidently handling the exam, you strengthen your belief in your abilities and reduce anxiety.

How to Practice:

1. **Close Your Eyes:**

   - Find a quiet spot, close your eyes, and take a few deep breaths.

2. **Visualize the Exam Process:**

   - Picture yourself walking into the exam room feeling calm and prepared.
   - Imagine reading each question with clarity, understand-

ing it fully, and answering confidently.

3. **See Yourself Succeeding:**

    - Visualize the moment you complete the exam with a sense of accomplishment and peace, knowing you've done your best.

Example: While waiting for the exam to start, take a minute to visualize yourself succeeding. Picture every detail, from your steady breathing and focused concentration to the satisfaction of completing the test.

Inspirational Verse:

Philippians 4:6-7—"Do not be anxious about anything, but in every situation, by prayer and petition, with thanksgiving, present your requests to God. And the peace of God, which transcends all understanding, will guard your hearts and your minds in Christ Jesus."

This verse reminds you to bring your worries to God, trusting Him to provide peace and clarity. Let His presence calm your heart as you prepare to give your best effort.

Encouragement:

Spending a few minutes practicing relaxation techniques can significantly improve exam performance. Deep breaths and positive visualization are not just strategies—they're acts of self-care and faith. With a calm mind, a steady heart, and trust in your preparation, you're ready to succeed. Remember, you've worked hard for this moment, and you are capable of great things.

5. Use Test-Taking Strategies

Approaching the exam methodically can significantly improve your performance and ensure you make the most of your knowledge and preparation. By following proven strategies, you'll stay focused, manage your time effectively, and maintain confidence throughout the test.

Read Instructions Carefully

Why It Matters:

Understanding the directions ensures that you answer questions in the expected format and manner, avoiding unnecessary errors due to misinterpretation.

How to Apply:

- Take a moment to thoroughly read the instructions for each section.
- Look for specific details, such as whether multiple answers are allowed or how to format responses.

Example: Jane almost skipped an entire section because she didn't notice the instruction to scroll down. Pausing to review the directions saved her from losing critical points.

Pace Yourself

Why It Matters:

Proper pacing ensures you allocate enough time for all questions, reducing the risk of running out of time before completing the test.

How to Apply:

- Watch the clock to monitor your progress and modify your speed as necessary.
- If you encounter a challenging question, flag it and move on to the next. Revisiting difficult questions later prevents you from getting stuck.

Example: Mark decided to move on from a tough math question and returned to it later, finishing the rest of the test with time to spare.

Eliminate Distractors

Why It Matters:

Crossing out answers that are clearly incorrect increases your chances of selecting the correct option, even if you're unsure of the answer.

How to Apply:

- Look for options that don't align with the question or are obviously wrong.
- Focus on narrowing the choices to two or three possibilities, then select the best answer.

Example: Emily wasn't sure about the answer to a question but eliminated two distractors, improving her odds and choosing correctly.

Trust Your Instincts

Why It Matters:

Your first instinct is often based on your preparation and understanding. Overthinking can sometimes lead to unnecessary changes that lower accuracy.

How to Apply:

- Go with your initial answer unless you identify a clear mistake or recall new information that changes your choice.
- Avoid second-guessing yourself unnecessarily.

Example: Sarah made a spontaneous change to her answer, only to discover later that her initial choice was accurate. From then on, she trusted her instincts, improving her overall score.

Encouragement and Verse:

Approaching the exam with strategy and focus reflects your hard work and preparation. Trust in your abilities, lean on the skills you've developed, and remember this verse as your guide:

Proverbs 16:3—"Commit to the Lord whatever you do, and He will establish your plans."

Applying these strategies with faith and diligence will set you up for success. Stay steady, trust your preparation, and confidently tackle each question—you are ready for this!

6. Manage Breaks Wisely

Scheduled breaks during the exam are not just a pause—they're a vital opportunity to recharge your mind and body. Taking a moment to step away allows you to refocus, reduce stress, and maintain energy levels, ensuring you're ready to tackle the next part of the exam with clarity and confidence.

What to Do During Breaks

- **Stretch:**
    - Relieve physical tension by standing up, rolling your shoulders, or gently stretching your neck and arms. If possible, take a short walk around the designated break area.
    - **Why It Helps:** Movement increases blood flow, helping you feel more alert and reducing stiffness from sitting for long periods.
- **Snack and Hydrate:**
    - Refuel with light, healthy snacks such as granola bars, nuts, or fruit. Drink water to stay hydrated, but avoid overindulgence, which can make you feel sluggish.

    - **Why It Helps:** Stable energy prevents fatigue and ensures your mind stays sharp for the remainder of the test.

- **Recenter:**
    - Take a minute or two to practice deep breathing or recite a calming verse. This will help you quiet your mind and regain focus.
    - **Why It Helps:** A quick moment of mindfulness can help you reset emotionally, reduce anxiety, and restore confidence.

Example:

During her exam break, Sarah spent two minutes stretching, enjoyed a handful of almonds and a bottle of water, and quietly recited *Matthew 11:28* to herself. This routine helped her return to the test with a calm mind and renewed energy.

Inspirational Verse:

Matthew 11:28—"Come to me, all who labor and are heavy laden, and I will give you rest."

This verse reminds us to trust in God's provision of rest and renewal. Lean into His promise to refresh your spirit, even in moments of pressure or fatigue.

Encouragement:

Breaks are a gift—an opportunity to step back, breathe, and remind yourself that you are prepared and capable. Use them wisely to recharge both your mind and body, trusting that each pause brings you closer to completing the exam with focus and grace. You've got this!

7. Stay Positive Throughout the Exam

On exam day, your mindset can significantly impact your performance. Staying positive not only helps you remain calm and focused but also reinforces the confidence you need to succeed. By managing your thoughts and celebrating small victories, you can maintain a sense of control and optimism throughout the test.

Reframe Negative Thoughts

Why It Matters:

Negative thoughts can undermine your confidence and create unnecessary stress. By replacing them with positive affirmations, you empower yourself to approach the exam with clarity and determination.

How to Apply:

- Replace self-doubt with empowering thoughts.
  - Instead of "I can't do this," say, "I am prepared and capable."
  - Instead of "This question is too hard," think, "I'll do my best and move on if needed."
- Focus on one question at a time. Avoid worrying about the entire exam or what's ahead—just tackle what's in front of you.

Example:

When Sarah felt overwhelmed by a tricky question, she reminded herself, "I've prepared for this. I'll answer what I can and come back if needed." This mindset kept her calm and focused.

Celebrate Small Wins

Why It Matters:

Acknowledging your achievements during the exam—even small

ones—helps you stay motivated and focused. Recognizing progress reinforces your confidence and prevents frustration from taking over.

How to Apply:

- Celebrate completing a difficult question or successfully recalling information.
- Congratulate yourself for staying calm under pressure or for effectively using a test-taking strategy.

Example:

After solving a particularly challenging math problem, Mark silently acknowledged his effort, thinking, "That was tough, but I handled it." This small celebration boosted his confidence for the next question.

Inspirational Verse:

Philippians 4:13—"I can do all things through Him who strengthens me."

This verse reminds you to draw strength from your faith, trusting that God has equipped you to face challenges with courage and grace.

Encouragement:

Staying positive during the exam is as much about faith as it is about preparation. Trust in the hard work you've put in and in the God who strengthens you. Every question you answer is a step forward—acknowledge your progress, focus on the present, and approach each moment with confidence. You've got this!

8. Review Answers Before Submitting

Taking time to review your answers before submitting the exam is a critical step that can make a big difference in your final performance. Revisiting flagged questions and double-checking your work allows you to catch errors, correct mistakes, and ensure you've given each question your best effort.

Revisit Flagged Questions

Why It Matters:

Flagged questions often require more thought or a second look. Approaching them with a fresh perspective can provide clarity and lead to a better answer.

How to Apply:

- Return to any flagged questions and carefully reread them, considering whether additional insights or a different approach might help.
- Avoid overthinking your original answer, but if you identify a clear mistake or recall new information, don't hesitate to change it.

Example:

Emma flagged a question involving a confusing calculation. When she revisited it, a second look helped her realize her initial error, allowing her to correct it and gain confidence in her answer.

Double-Check Data

Why It Matters:

Numerical answers, calculations, or data-based responses can easily contain small errors. Reviewing these ensures your answers align with the question requirements and are free of typos or missteps.

How to Apply:

- Verify that numerical answers are calculated correctly and formatted as required (e.g., decimal points, units).
- Ensure that any charts, graphs, or data points used to answer questions match the original information provided in the exam.

Example:

Before submitting, John double-checked a series of calculations and realized he had misread a unit in one of the questions. Correcting it earned him valuable points.

Encouragement and Verse:

Your review of your answers reflects the diligence and focus you've put into your preparation. Trust in your instincts, take a steady approach, and let your hard work shine through in your final submission.

Psalm 37:5—"Commit your way to the Lord; trust in Him, and He will act."

By carefully reviewing your work with patience and trust, you're ensuring that your effort and preparation are fully reflected in your results. You've done the work—now finish strong!

9. Pray or Meditate Before and After

Connecting spiritually before and after the exam can provide a deep sense of comfort, clarity, and strength. Prayer or meditation helps calm your nerves, focus your mind, and remind you that you are not alone in this journey. Trusting in God or grounding yourself through reflection allows you to approach the exam with confidence and leave it in peace.

Before the Exam

Why It Matters:

Starting your exam with prayer or meditation sets the tone for the day. It invites peace into your heart, asks for guidance, and reminds you to trust in the preparation you've done.

What to Do:

- Take a quiet moment to center yourself. Close your eyes, take a few deep breaths, and reflect on your hard work and dedication.

- Ask for wisdom, focus, and peace as you begin the test.

Prayer Example:

"Lord, thank You for guiding me through this journey and giving me the strength to prepare. I ask for clarity, focus, and confidence as I take this exam. Help me to trust in the knowledge You've helped me gain and to approach this moment with a calm heart. Amen."

After the Exam

- **Why It Matters:**
  After completing the test, taking time to reflect and pray helps you release any lingering anxiety and trust God with the results. This moment allows you to express gratitude for your effort and find peace in knowing that you've done your best.

What to Do:

- Pause to reflect on your efforts and acknowledge the completion of this important step.
- Pray for trust in God's plan for your success and for patience as you await the results.

Prayer Example:

"Father, I thank You for being with me during this exam and giving me the strength to complete it. I trust in Your plan for my success and know that the results are in Your hands. Help me to rest in peace and gratitude, knowing I've done my best. Amen."

Inspirational Verse:

Philippians 4:6-7—"Do not be anxious about anything, but in every situation, by prayer and petition, with thanksgiving, present your requests to God. And the peace of God, which transcends all understanding, will guard your hearts and your minds in Christ Jesus."

Encouragement:

Prayer and meditation are powerful tools for finding strength, clarity, and peace before and after your exam. Trust that your preparation, combined with faith, has equipped you for success. No matter what happens, a higher plan is there to support and direct you. You've given your best effort—rest in that assurance.

Final Thought

The day of your exam is not just about demonstrating your knowledge—it's a culmination of your preparation, your resilience, and your faith. It's about trusting the work you've done, managing your mindset, and leaning on the strength and guidance that God provides.

As you step into the testing room, remind yourself of the journey that has brought you here. You've put in the time, the effort, and the prayer. Now it's your moment to shine. Whether through careful planning, relaxation techniques, or spiritual grounding, you've equipped yourself with the tools to succeed.

Breathe deeply, place your trust in your preparation, and walk confidently, knowing that God's plans for you are filled with hope and a bright future.

Jeremiah 29:11—"For I know the plans I have for you, declares the Lord, plans for welfare and not for evil, to give you a future and a hope."

This verse reminds you that your efforts are part of a bigger plan, one designed for your success and well-being. You are not alone in this journey; God is with you every step of the way.

You've done your part. Now it's time to let your light shine. You've got this!

CHAPTER 9

DETAILED STUDY PLAN FOR THE AGPCNP EXAM

"For which of you, desiring to build a tower, does not first sit down and count the cost, whether he has enough to complete it?"
Luke 14:28

This 8-week study plan will guide you through the key topics and skills required to succeed on the AGPCNP exam. It provides weekly goals, curated resources, and practical study tips to help you establish a strong knowledge base, develop test-taking strategies, and approach the exam confidently.

Week 1-2: Health Promotion & Disease Prevention Overview

Goals:

- Learn about screening guidelines, vaccinations, and health counseling.
- Focus on age-specific recommendations for adults and older adults.

Topics:

- USPSTF guidelines (e.g., mammograms, colonoscopies, DEXA scans).
- Immunization schedules (e.g., flu, shingles, pneumonia).
- Lifestyle interventions (e.g., smoking cessation, exercise, nutrition).

Activities:

- Read Leik's Adult-Gerontology Nurse Practitioner Certification Intensive Review, specifically focusing on the chapters related to Health Promotion.
- Create a chart detailing age-based screening and immunization schedules for better organization and reference.

- Take practice quizzes on prevention strategies from:
    - ANCC Practice Resources.
    - BoardVitals AGNP Practice Questions.

Study Tips:

- Dedicate time each day to review screening guidelines. Break them into smaller sections (e.g., screenings for 40-60 years old, 60+).
- Use color-coded charts to distinguish between immunizations and screenings by age group, enhancing retention and clarity.
- Enhance your study by utilizing visual aids, such as the CDC's immunization schedules, to facilitate a better understanding of the content.

Example Question:

A 65-year-old male with no health complaints presents for a check-up. Which screenings and immunizations should be recommended for this patient?

- **Answer:** Influenza vaccine, pneumococcal vaccine, shingles vaccine, colonoscopy (if not done in the last 10 years).

Week 3-4: Assessment & Diagnosis

Goals:

- Master history taking, physical exams, and interpretation of lab/diagnostic tests.
- Identify common conditions in primary care for adults and geriatrics.

Topics:

- Comprehensive adult and geriatric assessments.
- Diagnostic imaging and lab tests (e.g., CBC, CMP, lipid panels, urinalysis).
- Symptom-based differential diagnosis (e.g., fatigue, chest pain, back pain).

Activities:

- Study *Fitzgerald's Nurse Practitioner Certification Exam and Practice Preparation* (Chapters on diagnostics and common presentations).
- Practice SOAP note writing for common conditions.
- Take practice tests from:
    - Exam Edge AGNP Tests.

- Barkley Diagnostic Exams.

Study Tips:

- To better understand, focus on one body system at a time (e.g., cardiovascular, endocrine, or musculoskeletal).
- Practice interpreting lab results with real-life scenarios or mock cases.
- Record yourself explaining diagnostic pathways to solidify your thought process.

Example Question:

A 55-year-old presents with fatigue and weight gain. Lab results show TSH is elevated. What is the diagnosis, and what is the initial treatment plan for this patient?

- **Answer:** Hypothyroidism; start levothyroxine.

Week 5-6: Plan of Care

Goals:

- Develop treatment plans, including pharmacological and non-pharmacological interventions.
- Learn about chronic disease management (e.g., diabetes, hy-

pertension, COPD).

Topics:

- Pharmacology (medications, side effects, interactions).
- Chronic conditions and management guidelines (e.g., ADA, AHA).
- Referral and collaborative care.

Activities:

- Use *Leik's Review* for concise disease management summaries.
- Watch pharmacology lectures on Nurse Practitioner Pharmacology YouTube Channels for comprehensive learning.
- Practice test-taking with clinical scenario questions:
    - Pocket Prep App.
    - Quizlet Flashcards.

Study Tips:

- Group similar medications (e.g., ACE inhibitors, beta-blockers) and compare their uses, side effects, and contraindications.

- Practice writing out treatment plans for common chronic conditions to strengthen recall.

- Consider joining Facebook groups like the AGNP Certification Study Group to receive support, share resources, and gain diverse perspectives. These platforms can enhance your learning by providing diverse perspectives and explanations. Members often share study tips, resources, and practice questions, offering fresh insights into complex topics. Additionally, study groups create a sense of community, providing emotional support and encouragement during your preparation journey.

Example Question:

What is the first-line treatment for hypertension in an older adult with diabetes?

- **Answer:** ACE inhibitors or ARBs (per ADA guidelines).

Week 7: Review and Practice

Goals:

- Solidify knowledge and improve speed in answering questions.

- Identify weak areas and reinforce them.

Activities:

- Review notes, flashcards, charts, and other study materials from previous weeks for a thorough revision.
- Take a full-length practice test (3-4 hours) to simulate exam conditions:
    - ANCC Practice Test.
    - Barkley Full-Length Practice Exam.

Study Tips:

- Mimic test-day conditions: set a timer, find a quiet space, and avoid distractions.
- Focus on pacing yourself to ensure you're answering questions within the allotted time.
- Use practice test results to identify weak areas and prioritize those for additional review.

Example Question:

A 70-year-old female has a history of osteoporosis and is on alendronate. What specific parameters should be monitored regularly for this patient?

- **Answer:** Calcium, vitamin D levels, and DEXA scans every 2 years.

Week 8: Final Review

Goals:

- Focus on test-taking strategies and exam readiness.
- Reduce anxiety and build confidence.

Activities:

- Review "Exam Tips" from *Leik's Review* (test-taking strategies and pitfalls).
- Revisit your weak topics and take focused practice quizzes.
- Relax the day before the exam—avoid last-minute cramming.

Study Tips:

- Practice deep breathing exercises to calm pre-exam nerves.
- Review key points with high-yield summaries or flashcards.
- Prepare all materials (ID, admission ticket, snacks) the night before to avoid last-minute stress.

Additional Tools and Resources

Mobile Apps:

- **Pocket Prep:** Practice questions and quizzes.
- **UWorld:** Comprehensive question bank with rationales.

Websites:

- CDC Immunization Schedulefor reference on immunization timing.
- USPSTF Guidelinesfor preventive service recommendations.

Study Groups:

- Join Facebook groups like "AGNP Certification Study Group" for support and shared resources.

Videos:

- *RegisteredNurseRN YouTube Channel* for quick topic reviews.

By following this comprehensive study plan, you will cover essential topics effectively, practice efficiently, and approach the AGPCNP exam with confidence.

REFERENCES

American Diabetes Association (ADA): https://diabetes.org/
American Cancer Society (ACS): https://www.cancer.org/
American Heart Association (AHA): https://www.heart.org/
Centers for Disease Controls and Prevention (CDC) : cdc.gov

National Library of Medicine: Screening to Prevent Osteoporotic Fractures: An Evidence Review for the U.S. Preventive Services Task Force [Internet]. https://www.ncbi.nlm.nih.gov/books/NBK532080/table/table1/#:~:text=Recommend%20BMD%20testing%20by%20DXA,frequent%20than%20every%202%20years

The American College of Obstetricians and Gynecologists: https://www.acog.org/

U.S. Preventive Services Task Force (USPSTF): https://www.uspreventiveservicestaskforce.org/uspstf/

www.ingramcontent.com/pod-product-compliance
Lightning Source LLC
La Vergne TN
LVHW052322200926
848481LV00002B/646

* 9 7 9 8 2 3 0 5 4 0 7 7 9 *